ASTHMA

The Complete Guide for Sufferers and Carers

GW00686206

ASTHMA

The Complete Guide for Sufferers and Carers

DR DERYK WILLIAMS,
ANNA WILLIAMS AND LAURA CROKER

PIATKUS

AUTHORS' NOTE

Throughout the book when several drug names occur together, we have listed them alphabetically and thus without expressing a preference.

> This book is dedicated to Bill Williams
> 1931–1979

First published in 1996 by
Judy Piatkus (Publishers) Ltd
5 Windmill Street, London W1P 1HF

The moral right of the authors has been asserted

A catalogue record for this book
is available from the British Library

ISBN 0–7499–1606–0 pbk

Designed by Sue Ryall
Artworks by One-Eleven Line-Art

Set in 11/13 pt Plantin by Phoenix Photosetting, Chatham, Kent
Printed and bound in Great Britain by
Mackays of Chatham PLC, Chatham, Kent

CONTENTS

ACKNOWLEDGEMENTS

We are grateful for the help given to us by the following people and organisations:

Mike Andrews, Toby Anstis, Astra Pharmaceuticals Ltd, Greta Barnes and the Asthma Training Centre, Mark Britton, Teresa Chris, Patrick Farrell, Mike Gardner, Mike Garrett, Glaxo Wellcome, Annabel Hancock and Halstead Preparatory School, Karen MacLeod, Dr John Moore-Gillon and The British Lung Foundation, Adrian Moorhouse OBE, Claire Nixon of the National Asthma Campaign's Asthma Helpline team, Janice Richardson and Pilgrims School, Michele Verroken, Fiona Walsh.

We would also particularly like to thank our friends and families for all their support and encouragement, especially David, Jessica, Tessa, Daniella, Daisy, Olivia and Isabella.

1

THE FACTS ABOUT
ASTHMA

You probably know someone who has asthma. You may be looking after an asthmatic child or elderly person. Perhaps you have a close friend or relative who is suffering from the disease. Perhaps you suffer from asthma yourself.

The first thing to realise is that you do not have to be thwarted by asthma. It can be managed and, most importantly, it need not spoil your life. To tackle asthma you have to know the facts, and what you can do yourself. This book gives you the information you need to take control.

Why Is Asthma More Common In Certain Countries?

There are now three million known asthmatics in Britain – 6 per cent of the population. Of these, one million are children. Asthma does not recognise boundaries. It cuts across social divides; it is rife in cities and in the countryside, it is present in areas of clean and polluted air; it is a disease of male and female, old and young.

Most of Western Europe and North America have the same proportions of diagnosed asthmatics as Britain. New

Zealand tops the league table, with 17 per cent of the population diagnosed as asthmatic, followed by Australia at 13 per cent. The significant point is that asthma is far less common in the developing world. In India and Africa only about 3 per cent of the population has asthma. Of these 3 per cent, most are living in cities.

Does this mean that people in the developed world are genetically more likely to develop asthma? Or are there factors in the environment, or in the way people live in the developed world, which cause them to develop asthma?

Some years ago a fascinating natural experiment occurred. The entire population of the Tokelau Islands in the South Pacific had to be moved to New Zealand following severe hurricane damage on the Islands. On the Tokelau Islands, asthma was almost unknown. However, after moving to New Zealand, many of the islanders developed asthma, and it was a particularly widespread problem among the children. This suggests that it is not so much genetic differences between populations that are important in the development of asthma, as the environment in which people live.

Although most of us have no choice about the environment in which we find ourselves, it is possible to make changes which improve that environment for asthmatics. This book gives simple, practical advice on how to do this.

Why Do People Die Of Asthma?

Twenty years ago relatively few people were diagnosed as asthmatics, and it was certainly not generally known that people died from the disease. Asthma claims about 2,000 lives in Britain annually, and about 40 of these will be children. The real tragedy is that nearly all these deaths are avoidable.

So why do so many people die of asthma? The fact is that 50 per cent of asthmatics are receiving inadequate medication from their doctors, which leaves them open to the possibility of a life-threatening asthma attack. Another 50 per cent do not take their medication properly, and so are also at risk of having a severe attack. This book therefore places particular emphasis on the importance of correct diagnosis and medication.

Another reason is that, as a life-threatening asthma attack develops, its severity can be misjudged. This leads to a crucial delay in the asthmatic receiving life-saving medical help. Doctors, carers and asthmatics themselves can be responsible for these errors of judgement. This book explains how to recognise a life-threatening asthma attack and what you can do about it.

Why Is Proper Treatment So Important?

Asthma that is undiagnosed, or under-treated, makes people ill. A child suffering from undiagnosed asthma can lose up to 50 days of schooling a year. If his asthma is keeping him awake at night he will be tired the next day, and will inevitably struggle in any activity requiring physical exertion. Likewise, undiagnosed adults will be forced to take time off work, resulting in lost productivity and increased sickness and invalidity benefit claims. Correct asthma management improves the quality of life for both children and adults as well as making economic sense.

These days asthma is discussed everywhere: on television, radio and in the newspapers; in our schools, hospitals and doctors' waiting rooms; at work and social events. As a result of all this public debate, asthma myths and misunderstandings abound, and a person facing asthma for the first time may find it difficult to know what to believe.

This book gives you the facts about asthma. It shows how carers and sufferers can live normal lives in spite of their asthma and how, by using commonsense and taking their medication as prescribed, asthmatics can help themselves to be well and achieve their full potential.

Twenty-six-year-old **Toby Anstis** is a presenter for BBC Television. He is energetic, confident and a rising star. This is his asthma story:

About five years ago we moved to an older house. My breathing became a little wheezy. The doctor thought it might be a chest infection, but after being lent a Ventolin inhaler I found the symptoms were alleviated. Consequently I was diagnosed as being a mild asthmatic. A mixture of house dust mites, old house dust and cat fur were found to be the triggers for my asthma.

I reckon that each day I have to use my blue inhaler once or twice, and that seems to keep the asthma at bay.

Having mentioned the combination of triggers, I must point out a problem situation which happened at work, at the BBC Television Centre. It was a very warm, humid, pollen-full day, and I was learning to rollerblade for a live item on Children's BBC. After about twenty minutes I felt my chest tighten, and spontaneous wheezing began. It got worse quickly and I had to bolt up to the office, where I puffed several times on my inhaler. Since then I have always kept my inhaler in my jeans pocket, just in case.

I certainly find that two good aerobic workouts and one circuit training session each week keep the lungs well exercised and supple. I believe this is helping to prevent the likelihood of an attack. (Although I do not underestimate the potential danger asthma can breathe into the lives of sufferers.)

My life as a mild asthmatic is fulfilling and energetic. You can beat asthma if you put your mind and body to it!

FOOTNOTE: *As we will see later, people like Toby who need to use their blue reliever inhaler daily, are now advised to use regular preventative treatment.*

2

WHAT IS ASTHMA?

The word 'asthma' is derived from the Greek word *az-ma* which means 'to breathe hard'. Features that are typical of asthma include wheezing while breathing out (expiring), feeling short of breath, tightness in the chest, and a persistent cough. These features combine to make 'breathing hard'. First of all let's look at how the lungs work, and then at what happens in the lungs to cause asthma.

How The Lungs Work

The lungs are constructed like an upside-down tree, with the trunk (trachea) branching out into a series of medium-sized branches (bronchi) that split into smaller branches and twigs (bronchioles). The trachea, bronchi and bronchioles are collectively known as the airways and are encased in a layer of muscle. At the end of the bronchioles are vast numbers of air-filled sacs (alveoli) that resemble tiny bunches of grapes (see diagram on p. 6).

The lungs deliver oxygen (O_2) molecules to the alveoli. These molecules then pass through the walls of the alveoli and the adjacent blood vessels and thus into the bloodstream. Here O_2 molecules combine with red blood cells in order to be transported to every cell in the body as an essential fuel for metabolism (see p. 7). O_2 molecules are combined with

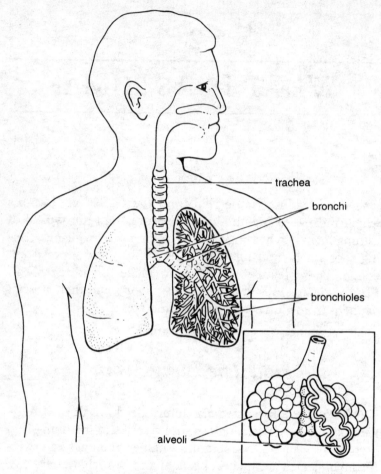

The inside of the lungs

carbon atoms during metabolism, forming the waste product carbon dioxide (CO_2). CO_2 is delivered back to the lungs in the bloodstream, via the walls of the blood vessels and alveoli, to be expelled by the lungs when we breathe out.

The branching structure of the lungs, together with all the air-filled sacs (alveoli), creates an enormous surface area to aid the transfer of O_2 and CO_2 between the lungs and the bloodstream. In an average adult male, this surface area is equivalent to two tennis courts!

> ## WHAT IS METABOLISM?
>
> Every minute of the day there are millions of chemical reactions going on inside our bodies. These reactions generate growth, provide energy and get rid of waste products. The body's metabolism is the sum total of these chemical reactions and O_2 is an essential fuel for all of them.

Why Is 'Breathing Hard' With Asthma?

An asthma attack occurs when the small and medium-sized airways get inflamed. This means that they become red and swollen, which narrows the space inside them. It is just the same as when you spill very hot water onto your arm. This triggers swelling and redness, known as inflammation. (The word inflammation is from the Latin word *inflammare* which means 'to flame within'.)

Inside the lungs, hostile factors (such as viruses or pollutants) cause the inner layer (lining) of the airways to become inflamed in much the same way. The problem within the lungs is that the outside of an airway is fairly rigid. Because of this, the red and swollen lining of the airway can only expand into the hollow part (lumen) of the airway. The inflammation causes the encasing muscle to contract, further narrowing the airway and causing breathing to become increasingly hard. When the lumen becomes narrowed, it is difficult for O_2 to reach the bloodstream, and for CO_2 to be removed (see diagram on p. 8).

Asthma is a dangerous condition because it can stop the continuous supply of oxygen which the body needs as a basic fuel for the metabolism of every cell.

7

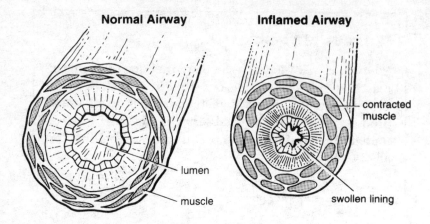

The inside of a normal and an inflamed airway

WHY DO ASTHMATICS WHEEZE WHEN BREATHING OUT?

Usually the wheeze in asthma occurs while the person breathes out (expiration). While the person breathes in (inspiration), the chest expands, opening up the airways, allowing air to flow into the lungs. During expiration, the chest contracts, pushing air out of the lungs, but at the same time causing the airways to become narrower. Wheezing is rather like whistling; pushing air through pursed lips produces a sound similar to a wheeze. For a healthy person, inspiration and expiration last about the same length of time, but during an asthma attack expiration takes longer because the person is trying to squeeze the air through a narrowed airway.

The Inflammatory Response

The inflammatory response (see p. 10) is designed to protect the body from hostile factors in the environment. Examples of factors that are hostile to everybody's lungs, whether or not they are asthmatic, are the cold virus or pollutants in the atmosphere. The hostile factor is inhaled into the lungs and sticks to the surface of the airways. Your body uses the inflammatory response to break down and remove these hostile factors.

For an inflammatory response to occur, the body needs white blood cells (as opposed to the red blood cells that transport O_2), and powerful chemicals (inflammatory mediators). These circulate in the bloodstream, and pass through blood vessel walls and between cells.

The inflammatory response starts when the blood vessels surrounding the hostile factor become wider (dilate). They increase the supply of blood in order to rush as many white blood cells and inflammatory mediators to the area as possible. The walls of the blood vessels then become leaky, allowing the white blood cells and inflammatory mediators to engulf the hostile factor. Here, the white blood cells and inflammatory mediators interact to break down and remove the hostile factor and so combat the threat to the body. The redness is caused by the dilation of the blood vessels, and the swelling is caused by the blood vessels becoming leaky. Once the hostile factor has been made harmless, the inflammation quickly dies down.

INFLAMMATION AND ASTHMA

Inflammation is an essential part of the functioning of a healthy lung. Minute areas of inflammation occur thousands of times every day in our lungs in order to combat hostile factors such as the viruses, bacteria and pollutants to which we

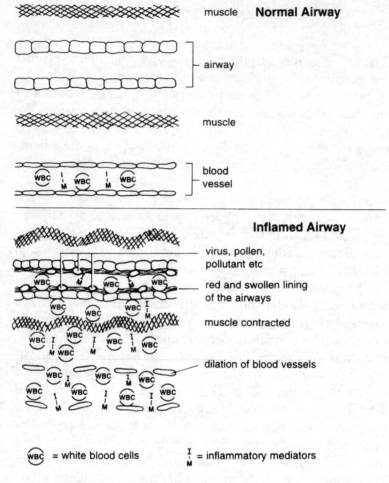

Normal Airway

muscle

airway

muscle

blood vessel

WBC   WBC   WBC

Inflamed Airway

— virus, pollen, pollutant etc

— red and swollen lining of the airways

muscle contracted

— dilation of blood vessels

WBC = white blood cells $\frac{I}{M}$ = inflammatory mediators

The inflammatory response

are exposed. None of this activity produces any symptoms, and we are totally unaware of it.

However asthmatics massively over-react (hyper-react) to such hostile factors, aggravating inflammation throughout the small and medium-sized airways in their lungs. An acute asthma attack occurs when the airways get so inflamed and narrow that very little air can get through.

To recap then, the airways of asthmatics are *super-primed*, massively over-reacting to hostile factors in the environment, causing the airways to become narrowed, and interfering with the crucial supply of O_2 to the body.

3

WHAT CAUSES ASTHMA?

Genetic Factors

The tendency to develop asthma is passed down through families. People with asthma, or people who could develop asthma at any time, carry this tendency in their genes. About 30 per cent of the population has an underlying tendency to develop asthma, but only about half of these people actually go on to suffer with the disease.

WHAT IS A GENE?

Genes determine your physical characteristics – your height, eye colour, hair colour, and so on. Millions of genes are combined in chains to form chromosomes and every cell in your body has 46 chromosomes (apart from sperm and eggs which have half this number). Half your genes come from your mother and the other half from your father.

Most of the traits we inherit are determined by combinations of genes. The stronger the combination of genes, the more prominent the trait. For example, if all the genes you have inherited from your parents are for a tall person, then you will be tall. If, on the other hand, you have inherited genes for a small person from your mother and genes for a tall person from your father, then you will most probably be somewhere between the two. Likewise, if your father has brown hair and your mother blonde hair, your eventual hair colour may be light brown (or possibly blonde or dark brown).

There are, however, two different types of inherited traits. Firstly, there are the *fixed* traits which are not influenced by the environment. For example, your hair colour will be the same regardless of how you interact with the environment. Secondly, there are *variable* traits which can be modified by your environment. For instance, although your potential height is determined by the genes you have inherited from your parents, you will only reach that height if your inter-action with the environment gives you access to a good diet.

The tendency to develop asthma works in a similar way. It is the combination of your genes and your interaction with the environment that determines whether you will develop asthma, and how severe the asthma will be. Having two severely asthmatic parents may mean that asthma will develop very readily, be provoked by many factors in the environment, and be quite severe. On the other hand, a person with one mildly asthmatic parent may never develop asthma or only develop it in response to specific factors.

Asthma Provoking Factors

An asthma sufferer may have mild symptoms for many years, and then suddenly develop an acute asthma attack, usually in response to a provoking factor in the environment. There are two main types of asthma provoking factors, *irritants* and *allergens*. We all encounter irritants and allergens in our daily lives, but it can sometimes be difficult to distinguish between them.

ALLERGENS

An allergic response occurs when the body mistakenly identifies the allergen as a hostile factor, and responds with *inappropriate* inflammation. For example, certain people are allergic to plasters; whenever they put on a plaster they get redness and blisters within a few hours. Although the plaster is quite harmless, the body mistakenly identifies it as a hostile factor and responds with inappropriate inflammation. In this case the plaster is an allergen.

In relation to asthma, grass pollen is a common allergen. Pollen is quite harmless to normal lungs but in asthma sufferers who are allergic to pollen it will cause an inappropriate inflammatory reaction, resulting in asthma symptoms.

THE ATOPIC TENDENCY

The genes that give a person an underlying tendency to develop asthma are the same genes that make them likely to suffer from other allergy problems: this is known as the atopic tendency. The two conditions that are most closely associated with asthma in this way are eczema and hayfever. (For more on this, see Chapter 14.)

IRRITANTS

An example of an irritant would be a stinging nettle. If you are unlucky and brush against a nettle, a chemical is released that damages your body and so your body defends itself with an *appropriate* inflammatory response.

There are irritants in our environment, such as cigarette

smoke or oxide of nitrogen (NO_x) from car exhaust, that affect the airways of both asthmatics and non-asthmatics. These irritants cause mild inflammatory reactions even in normal lungs. However in an asthma sufferer they may cause the underlying inflammation in the lining of the airways to flare up.

Initiators Of Asthma

Various provoking factors, either allergens or irritants, can cause an asthma sufferer's first asthma attack. We will call the factor that causes this first attack an initiator of asthma. Once an asthma sufferer has experienced the first symptoms of asthma, any factor that provokes asthma symptoms, even if it happens to be the initiator of asthma, is called a *trigger provoking factor*. The first asthma attack usually occurs during childhood, but may not occur until adulthood. From this point on, the inflammatory mechanism is unstable, or *primed*.

It is sometimes said that if a doctor is uncertain of the cause of an illness he or she will always blame a virus. However recent asthma research shows that 80 per cent of initial bouts of asthma *are* actually caused by viruses. The most common initiator of asthma is the rhinovirus, which is responsible for coughs and colds. Of the remaining 20 per cent of initial bouts of asthma, the most frequent culprits are cigarette smoke, the house dust mite, pollen and possibly pollution. However almost any environmental allergen or irritant can be responsible.

Triggers Of Asthma

Any asthma provoking factor that aggravates established asthma is called a trigger provoking factor, or simply a trigger. In our environment there is a very wide range of triggers. An

CAN I HELP PREVENT MY CHILD FROM DEVELOPING ASTHMA?

The most frequent initiator of asthma is the rhinovirus which causes the common cold. It is not possible to prevent your child from being exposed to this virus. However there are some other points that may usefully be considered:

- In any household, but particularly in a household with asthma, it is crucial that there is no cigarette smoke in the house. **Children living in a house with parents who smoke are twice as likely to develop asthma as children living in a non-smoking household. Smoking during pregnancy also increases the likelihood of a child developing asthma.**

- It may also help to try to reduce the allergens that an infant is exposed to in the first three months of life. This means keeping the amount of dust in the household, and also the exposure to pets, to a minimum.

- Breast-feeding does not appear to have any influence on whether or not a baby develops asthma. However breast-fed infants are less likely to develop eczema.

asthma sufferer may be sensitive to just one trigger that can be readily identified and easily avoided, such as cigarette smoke. Other asthma sufferers may be sensitive to many triggers. For example, apart from environmental factors, asthma can be triggered by strong emotions, both pleasant and unpleasant; stress; various medicines, either prescribed by your doctor or bought over the counter; and even different foods.

Irritants

VIRUSES

As we have seen, the rhinovirus, which causes coughs and colds, is the most common trigger of asthma, particularly in children. Often the asthma sufferer is treated with antibiotics for the cough and cold, and the asthma symptoms are overlooked. This is one of the major reasons for asthma remaining undiagnosed in so many people.

EXERCISE

Exercise is one of the most common triggers of asthma, affecting about 90 per cent of asthmatics. During exercise, there is a great increase in the amount of air that passes in and out of the lungs. This dries the lining of the airways, causing irritation and triggering asthma.

CIGARETTE SMOKE

This is one of the most potent triggers of asthma, and one of the few that can be avoided. If you have asthma yourself you should not smoke, fullstop. And you should never smoke if you have an asthmatic child in the home. To do so would be irresponsible.

ATMOSPHERIC POLLUTION

There are two main sources of atmospheric pollution: motor vehicle exhaust and power station emissions. Car exhaust contains a gas called oxides of nitrogen (NO_x) which is converted into an acid called nitric acid (HNO_3) when it reacts with the moisture on the surface of the airways. In a similar fashion, power station emissions contain a gas called sulphur dioxide, which forms an acid called sulphuric acid (H_2SO_4) when it reacts with the moisture on the surface of the airways. It is now thought that both of these acids irritate the airways, thus triggering asthma. (For more on atmospheric pollutants, see Chapter 13.)

COLD AIR

Going out of a warm house on a cold winter's day often triggers asthma. The blast of cold air dries out the airways, thus irritating the lungs and causing narrowing of the airways.

Allergens

HOUSE DUST MITES

These little bugs are number two in the league table for asthma triggers after the rhinovirus. In Britain and most other countries the most common species of the house dust mite is called *Dermatophagoides pteronyssinus*. In the USA the most common species is *Dermatophagoides farinae*. These charming little creatures live on and eat the flakes of skin we shed. They thrive in warm, damp bedding, especially where feathers are present. Most household dust is shedded human skin, so there is a rich feast available for them. It is the *faeces* of the mites rather than the mites themselves which trigger asthma.

POLLEN

Some asthma sufferers find that their asthma is triggered by specific pollens that are present in the environment at particular times of the year. For example, tree pollens are present in the spring, and grass pollens in the summer. Asthma which is only triggered by a specific pollen is called seasonal asthma. Of course pollens are also responsible for causing hayfever. Hayfever and asthma can occur together, but often only the hayfever is recognised. This is another reason for the under-diagnosis of asthma.

PETS

The beloved family pet can, unfortunately, be the cause of a great deal of suffering for an asthmatic. The pet that most frequently triggers asthma is the cat. The allergen is in the cat's saliva, which is transferred to its fur while grooming. Siamese and Burmese cats appear to produce the most potent asthma allergens. Dogs are also frequently responsible for triggering asthma. In dogs it is a mould growing on the dead flakes of skin (dander) that triggers asthma. However any pet with fur or feathers can trigger asthma.

Emotional Factors

Emotions can have a major influence on asthma. Feelings of anxiety, stress, or just being down and depressed can trigger an attack. As the attack develops, this in itself generates feelings of panic. The inability to function normally during the day may cause stress because of fear about the consequences of an asthma attack. It is not just unpleasant emotions that can trigger asthma: when we laugh we suddenly draw in large amounts of air that dry the airways, causing irritation and triggering asthma.

Medicines

ASPIRIN AND ASPIRIN-LIKE MEDICINES

About 5 per cent of asthmatics are sensitive to aspirin, and the majority of these people are elderly. A severe attack can be triggered about 20 minutes after taking an aspirin. If an asthmatic is sensitive to aspirin, they will also be sensitive to a range of aspirin-like medicines, such as medication used for treating arthritis. There are many other similar preparations, so if you know you have an aspirin sensitivity, always remind your doctor before he prescribes for you. Many medicines that you can buy without a prescription – including remedies for coughs, colds, headaches, and general pain-killers – may also contain aspirin. The box below lists some of the common preparations to avoid, but this is not a comprehensive list. To ensure your own safety, **always ask your pharmacist's advice before buying any medication**.

NON-PRESCRIPTION MEDICINES CONTAINING ASPIRIN OR ASPIRIN-LIKE MEDICATIONS

Anadin
Nurofen
Aspro
Alka Seltzer
Codis

Disprin
Veganin
Advil (available in the US only)
Bayer Buffered Aspirin Tablets (US only)

BETA BLOCKERS

Beta blockers cause the airways to constrict and should rarely be given to asthmatics. This type of medication acts in the opposite way to medications such as Ventolin which cause the airways to *open*. Beta blockers are usually prescribed for heart conditions such as high blood pressure, but can also be used to treat anxiety and panic. A doctor intending to prescribe beta blockers should always check whether or not a patient is asthmatic and all asthmatics should be aware of the danger associated with these drugs. If you are asthmatic and already taking a Beta blocker, see your doctor for advice.

BETA BLOCKING MEDICATION

Brand name	*Generic name*
Inderal	propranolol hydrochloride
Tenormin	atenolol
Sotacor	sotalol hydrochloride
Lopresor	metoprolol

Diet

In a small number of asthmatics certain foods seem to make asthma worse. The most commonly implicated foods are dairy products or eggs. If you suspect that your asthma is made worse by a particular food you can try an exclusion diet (described on p. 68) or skin prick testing (described on p. 67). The betel nut, *Areca catechu*, contains a chemical that causes the airways to contract in asthmatics. Betel nut chewing is particularly common within the Asian community. Although it does not affect all asthmatics, it is best avoided.

Food additives can also exacerbate asthma in a small number of asthmatics. These additives must be listed on the packaging, and in Europe the additives have been given numbers that must also appear on the packaging.

FOOD ADDITIVES

Monosodium glutamate (E621)

This is used as a flavour enhancer and is most commonly found in Chinese food. It may also be found in beefburgers, bacon, crisps, soups and many other food products.

Tartrazine (E102)

This is used to colour food (such as canned fruits, mustard, butter and margarine) and medicine capsules, yellow. About 50 per cent of asthmatics who are sensitive to aspirin will also be sensitive to tartrazine.

Sulphites and sulphur dioxide

These may be found in wines, beers, instant soups and synthetic orange drinks. Lettuce is often washed in metabisulphite to keep it looking fresh.

Benzoic acid (E210)

This is related to aspirin, and can be found in foods such as mushrooms, chocolate and yeast extract.

Chemicals

There are also many other, less common triggers. Just about any chemical that can be inhaled may trigger asthma. Even the propellant in metered dose inhalers can trigger asthma in a small percentage of people. If you notice, on a regular basis, a sudden deterioration in your asthma about *10* minutes after taking a puff of medication, you may need to change the type of inhaler you are using.

As it is impossible for asthma sufferers to avoid most of the factors that trigger their asthma, good asthma management is largely concerned with taking the correct medication in the dosage prescribed by your doctor. The next chapter explains the process of diagnosis and how your doctor decides what medication is appropriate for you.

4

DIAGNOSING ASTHMA

Diagnosing asthma is the first crucial step towards managing it successfully. As we have already seen, almost half of all asthmatics are not diagnosed and so do not receive treatment and continue to suffer needlessly. However there are also some cases where another condition is mistaken for asthma and the person receives unnecessary and inappropriate asthma treatment, so great care needs to be taken to ensure a correct diagnosis.

Conditions That May Be Mistaken For Asthma

HYPERVENTILATION

Asthma is *not* hyperventilation, although the conditions are often confused. Hyperventilation often occurs as the result of a panic attack which causes the person to breathe deeper and faster than usual. This breathing pattern is associated with a sensation of breathlessness, which may mislead people into thinking they are having an asthma attack. A useful distinguishing feature is that someone who is hyper-ventilating usually feels a tingling around the mouth and in the fingers.

CROUP

In children, croup can be confused with asthma. Croup is caused by a viral infection of the large upper airways, unlike asthma which is an inflammation of the smaller and medium-sized airways. Croup produces a harsh sound when the child is breathing in, and a barking cough akin to whooping cough. It is a condition that alarms parents, but it is not asthma.

BRONCHITIS AND EMPHYSEMA

Bronchitis and emphysema are chronic disorders of the medium-sized airways. These conditions affect an older age group, and nowadays are often the result of cigarette smoking. People with these conditions often have a chronic cough producing yellow phlegm, and have difficulty both breathing in and breathing out.

What Are The Distinguishing Features Of Asthma?

A big problem with recognising asthma is that it can co-exist with other conditions. Some people become panicky as an asthma attack develops, causing hyperventilation. The chronic infection and inflammation in bronchitis and emphysema can also result in features of asthma developing. However there are some distinguishing characteristics that you can look out for:

- In the airways of an asthmatic there is an ongoing inflammation, causing swelling of the lining of the airways and contraction of the encasing muscles, which results in the most readily identifiable feature of asthma – the expiratory wheeze. This can be provoked by any of the triggers discussed earlier.

- If a person has an expiratory wheeze they usually also complain of feeling short of breath, and have difficulty breathing in and out.

- Another common feature of asthma is a persistent cough that often produces yellow sputum, caused by the swollen lining of the airways provoking the cough reflex. The purpose of coughing is to clear the airways of the constriction caused by inflammation.

- These features of asthma – wheezing, coughing and shortness of breath – are typically worse at night and in the early morning.

- As the airways swell and the muscles contract, making the airways increasingly narrow, a feature called recession develops. This is a drawing in of the flesh between the ribs and above the sternum (breastbone), as the asthmatic expands his chest to suck air into his lungs. The more the asthmatic has to struggle to suck air into his lungs, the more noticeable the recession becomes.

- In mild asthma, with only minimal narrowing of the airways, the features may be quite subtle, and therefore easily missed or confused with other conditions. In children, there may be a persistent cough, but they may only complain of a tightness in the chest when the condition deteriorates. Because of the cough, children with mild asthma will often have been given many courses of antibiotics for coughs and colds. Adults, however, often think the shortness of breath after exercise is a result of not being fit, and do not realise that they may have exercise-induced asthma.

Diagnosing Asthma

If you recognise any of these features of asthma, the first step is to visit your doctor so that he can make a diagnosis and give appropriate asthma treatment. As asthma is a disease that tends to run down the generations, your doctor will need to know about your family medical history. He will ask about triggers, such as the presence of dust or animals, which may aggravate the breathing problems, and about when the problems are worse. This could be at different times of the day or night, autumn or spring, in cold temperatures, in polluted air or foggy weather. It is a good idea to keep a note of any times when you feel wheezy or short of breath, and tell your doctor when you see him.

In the surgery the doctor will refer back through your records, looking for recurrent coughs or colds (sometimes called chestiness), and repeated courses of antibiotics. These would indicate the likelihood of asthma.

The *story*, as doctors refer to this exploration of personal history, family history and assessment of the current situation, can account for about 90 per cent of a correct asthma diagnosis. The doctor will then examine you, particularly listening to your chest with his stethoscope to identify the expiratory wheeze. Once your doctor has a grasp of your story and has examined you, he may be satisfied that the story and examination are sufficient grounds on which to diagnose asthma. He will then be able to advise you how best to treat your asthma, and how to formulate an Asthma Management Plan (see Chapter 6).

Your doctor may also ask you to use a peak flow meter in order to assess how narrowed your airways are. You take in a deep breath and then breathe out as quickly as possible. The peak flow meter measures the speed at which air comes out of your lungs; the faster the air comes out, the less narrowing there will be of the airways. It is customary always to do three peak flows one after the other, and record the highest value.

If your doctor is unsure whether you have asthma, the peak flow readings will help to clarify the situation. Even if your doctor is sure you have asthma, they will help him to judge its severity.

Because asthma can wax and wane, sometimes just one peak flow measurement is not sufficient. In this case the doctor may ask you to take the peak flow meter home. Or he may prescribe a peak flow meter, so that you can take peak flow measurements and record them on a chart. The diagram below shows the correct way to use a peak flow meter. You will also need to record when you feel short of breath, and also your activities during the day to see if you can identify any triggers. The diagram on p. 30 shows a normal peak flow reading and a reading that demonstrates asthma. Features of the peak flow chart that are indicative of asthma are a 15 per cent difference between readings and drops in the peak flow readings in the morning (early morning dipping).

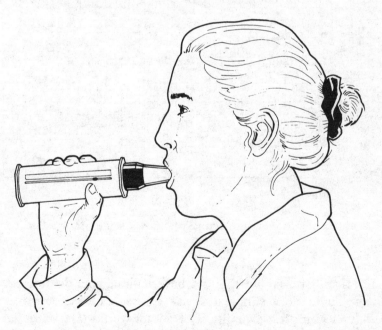

Using a peak flow meter

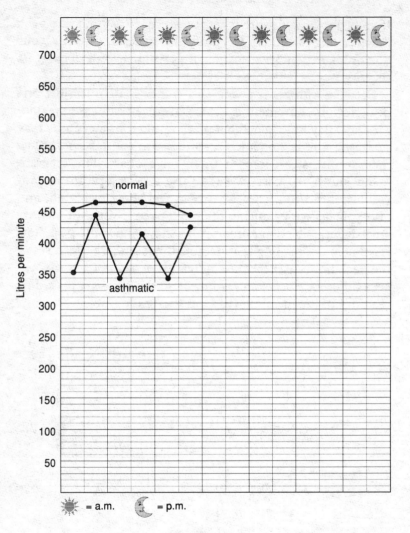

A peak flow chart showing a normal peak flow reading and an asthmatic peak flow reading

If it is still unclear whether you have asthma, your doctor may ask you to do a simple exercise test, as exercise provokes asthma in most asthmatics. The doctor would take an initial peak flow measurement and you would then exercise fairly vigorously for six minutes, stepping on and off a box. Five minutes after finishing the exercise, another peak flow measurement would be taken. A 15 per cent drop in peak flow would indicate a strong possibility of asthma.

Although asthma diagnosis can be a fairly lengthy and complex procedure, unfortunately some doctors are not particularly asthma-aware and may miss the diagnosis altogether. Even for the most asthma-aware doctor, the diagnosis can be difficult to make. This is because when a person comes to the surgery they are often not demonstrating any features of asthma, and many of the features of asthma overlap with those of other conditions such as coughs, colds, bronchitis and hyperventilation. Diagnosing asthma can be particularly difficult in young children who cannot relate their symptoms to a doctor and below 5 years of age, cannot use a peak flow meter to help the doctor make a diagnosis. The observations made by you, the parent, are crucial under these circumstances.

If your doctor has not diagnosed asthma but you think it is a strong possibility, you should start by discussing the issue in a polite but firm manner. All doctors know how easy it is to miss making a diagnosis of asthma, and will be grateful for your input.

If you feel that your doctor is still missing the diagnosis, first of all try and see another doctor in the same practice with an interest in asthma. This will often be stated in the practice leaflet, or he will be the doctor responsible for the asthma clinic (if there is one). Alternatively, insist on a specialist referral. Failing all these avenues, you are entitled to change to another practice. It will generally be known in the local community which doctors know about asthma, so ask around. Also, look for a practice with an asthma clinic, and see the doctor who is responsible for that clinic.

Anyone would be concerned when their doctor finally pronounces what sounds like a life sentence: 'You have asthma'. Since asthma is so common, you may know of people with severe or uncontrolled asthma. You may worry that you will come up against the difficulties they have. It is important to remember that the correct diagnosis is only the beginning; once the treatment is under way your asthma can be controlled, and need not place restrictions on your life.

5

TREATING ASTHMA

Reducing dust in the home, not smoking, eating a good diet and taking regular exercise may all help to control your asthma. But the mainstay of asthma management is regular medication. This is because the ongoing inflammation in the airways can never be cured. Even when you feel completely well and symptom-free, this low-grade inflammation will be waiting to flare up into an asthma attack. However, you *can* keep the inflammation under very good control using regular medication. The aim of asthma medication is to control the underlying inflammation, and enable asthma sufferers to lead a normal life.

There are a bewildering number of asthma medications available and, just to add to the confusion, each medication has two names – the *brand name* and the *generic name*. The generic name is the chemical compound, and the brand name is the name given to this chemical compound by a pharmaceutical company. To take an ordinary household example, vacuum cleaner is a generic name and Hoover is a brand name. In the same way, salbutamol is a generic (or chemical) name and Ventolin is the brand name of salbutamol. Because people tend to recognise brand names more easily, this book mainly refers to medications by their brand names first (with their generic names in brackets afterwards).

Brand Names And Generic Names

Understanding the distinction between brand names and generic names has become quite important. Doctors may sometimes change your prescription from a brand name to a generic name because generic drugs are cheaper than branded drugs. There should be no difference in effectiveness between the branded product and the generic product, but they will be produced by different manufacturers. If you notice any difference in effectiveness, you must let your doctor know immediately.

The two main types of asthma medication are *preventative* medication and *reliever* medication. There are also a number of other asthma medications used in addition to preventative and reliever medications, and these we will call *add-on* asthma medications.

Medicine for most conditions is taken by mouth. For example, if you have a throat infection, you take a course of antibiotic tablets. Quite high dosages of antibiotics are needed to treat a sore throat because the antibiotic has to be absorbed into the bloodstream via the intestines and is then passed around the body before reaching the throat. By this time, it has actually been diluted throughout the body. By contrast, asthma medication is usually inhaled, thus delivering the medication to the surface of the lungs where it is needed. This means that very low dosages can be used, greatly reducing the chances of any side-effects and enabling the medication to act more quickly. Certain asthma medications are taken in tablet or syrup form, either because there is no inhaled form of that medication, or because the person may find inhaling medication difficult.

Preventative Medication

Preventative inhalers are light brown, dark brown, maroon or orange, but never blue, this colour is reserved for reliever inhalers.

Preventative medication controls the underlying inflammation in the airways by preventing the blood vessels from dilating and becoming leaky. The inflammatory mediators and white blood cells can no longer flood into the airways, and so there is no redness, swelling or constriction of the muscle surrounding the airways. This medication is inhaled on a regular basis every day in order to keep the inflammation dampened down.

Usually, after an asthma sufferer has been taking preventative medication for a few days, the inflammation will come under control and he will start feeling a lot better. He may then make a very common mistake. Because he is feeling better, he may stop taking his preventative medication. The inflammation then begins to smoulder again, the airways become primed and unstable, and, given the appropriate trigger, will flare up into a full asthma attack. Preventative medication should *always* be taken, whether or not there are symptoms of asthma. **Never stop your preventative medication without medical advice.**

It is sometimes possible to stop taking asthma medication after you have been symptom-free for a long time, but this must only be under medical supervision. Children often seem to 'grow out' of asthma as they approach adolescence, particularly if their asthma has been quite mild. Their preventative medication is then reduced and, if they remain symptom-free, eventually stopped. However it is not unusual for asthma to flare up again in young adulthood, or even unpredictably during adolescence. It is rarely possible for adults to stop taking preventative medication.

The importance of always taking your medication

Fourteen-year-old Matthew's asthma required the use of a Ventolin inhaler three or four times a day. As this dosage is rather high, his doctor prescribed the preventer inhaler, Becotide, twice daily, rather than using the Ventolin so often.

Soon Matthew's asthma was well controlled, and his Ventolin use was cut right down. After three months on Becotide he was only using Ventolin once or twice a week.

After another three months on Becotide he hardly ever needed his Ventolin.

Without telling his mother or his doctor, Matthew decided that his asthma was cured, and so he stopped using his Becotide. Some time later he stayed with some friends and their pet cats, and soon began to wheeze. Matthew had not replaced his last empty Ventolin and so had no reliever, so he tried taking Becotide instead.

But Becotide does not improve asthma immediately, and Matthew's attack worsened. His mother took him to see his doctor, and he was given nebulised Ventolin. His attack subsided and he was able to breathe easier.

Matthew should not have stopped taking his preventer. He is asthmatic: the preventer can keep that condition under control, but it cannot cure it. He should always have a reliever inhaler at hand to deal with sudden wheezing. Taking a preventer when you need a reliever will not work, and may well lead to panic or tension which could even worsen an attack.

CORTICOSTEROIDS

Inhaled steroids are the most effective anti-inflammatory agents available. Examples of this type of medication are Becotide (beclomethasone), Flixotide (fluticasone), Pulmicort (budesonide), and, in the US, Azmacort (triamcinolone). Preventative medication is normally inhaled twice a day, which is particularly convenient because it means it does not have to be taken into school or into the workplace. More convenient still, Pulmicort can be taken just once a day.

The side-effects of steroids are a great source of concern to many people. The first point to emphasise is that the steroids used in asthma treatment are corticosteroids and not the anabolic, or body-building steroids, which have been subject to abuse. The second point is that only tiny amounts of steroid are absorbed into the body. Because steroid medication is nearly always inhaled, the medication is delivered straight to the surface of the lungs where it is needed, and very low dosages can be used.

As a parent, your main concern may be whether or not steroids will inhibit the growth of your child. However there is no evidence to suggest that children's growth is inhibited by normal steroid dosages. A few children have quite severe asthma that is difficult to control, and may therefore be on very high dosages of inhaled steroids. It is possible that there may be some inhibition of growth in these children. However they are most probably exchanging a centimetre of height for a reasonable quality of life, and quite possibly staying alive. Severe or untreated asthma can itself limit growth.

Other side-effects of steroids can include thrush in the mouth. Thrush is caused by a fungus called candida which produces redness and white spots in the mouth. It is associated with inhaled steroids because they inhibit the white cells that usually combat this fungus. Occasionally, inhaled steroids are associated with a certain degree of hoarseness but we don't really know why this is. Both these problems can be prevented by rinsing your mouth with water after inhalation. As a general rule it is therefore best to take inhaled steroids before brushing your teeth in the morning and at night. If the oral thrush or hoarseness persists, a spacer device can be helpful (see p. 47).

The all-important point to remember is that, used correctly under medical supervision for the treatment of asthma, **inhaled steroids are safe**.

CROMOGLYCATES

This type of drug is not a steroid but it *is* an anti-inflammatory agent. There are two brands available: Intal (cromoglycate) and a very similar drug called Tilade (nedocromil sodium). Intal is often used as the first choice anti-inflammatory medication in children because it has almost no side-effects. When Intal works, it is an effective medication, particularly in asthma triggered by allergies.

The problem with Intal is that it is not effective in all children, and therefore sometimes leaves children unwittingly exposed to asthma attacks. Steroids are therefore increasingly preferred as the first-choice preventative treatment for all children. Also, for reasons which are not entirely clear, Intal is not a particularly effective medication in adults.

Intal and Tilade are given four times a day by inhaler. Once the asthma is stabilised, this may then be reduced to three times a day. But this reduction must *only* take place under medical supervision.

Reliever Medication

Reliever medication is used to treat asthma symptoms, such as wheezing, coughing and shortness of breath. The medication relaxes the muscles surrounding the airways, and allows the airways to open up, or dilate, enabling the crucial supply of oxygen to get through to the blood stream. These types of medication are sometimes referred to as bronchodilators because they cause the bronchioles to open up. Reliever medications are usually inhaled, providing relief from asthma symptoms after about 15 seconds. However they are not anti-inflammatory, so they do not treat the underlying inflammation.

In the early stages of an asthma attack, or in very mild asthma, when the narrowing of the airways is mainly caused by the contraction of the surrounding muscle, reliever medication will give almost complete relief from asthma symptoms for about four to six hours. However, as an asthma attack develops and the lining of the airway gets more swollen, reliever medication becomes less effective. If there is incomplete relief of symptoms, or the symptoms return before four hours, this means your asthma is deteriorating dangerously and **urgent medical help should be sought**. In an emergency situation, you may need to use repeated doses of reliever medication. In fact, if you are having a severe asthma attack (and only under these circumstances) you may need to use a whole canister of reliever medication whilst awaiting medical assistance.

In the very mildest forms of asthma, the doctor may only prescribe reliever medication. However, if reliever medication is required more than once a day, you also need preventative medication. If you are already on preventative medication, and you need reliever medication more than once a day, this means that the amount of preventative medication needs to be increased. Preventative medication is really the mainstay of asthma treatment. Properly used, it should control the underlying inflammation so that reliever medication is rarely necessary.

Reliever medication is always blue. It should be carried with you at all times, and be used promptly to treat any asthma symptoms.

ADRENALINE-LIKE BRONCHODILATORS

Adrenaline is the natural chemical the body produces to open up the airways, in order to meet its greatly increased oxygen needs during times of crisis. Examples of this type of medication are Bricanyl (terbutaline) and Ventolin (salbutamol). These medications are similar to adrenaline, except that they act mainly on the airways and not on the rest of the body like adrenaline. They are nearly always inhaled, usually being prescribed as 'two puffs as required'. This means adrenaline-like inhalers can be used when necessary, but bearing in mind the considerations that have been described above.

These medications also come in tablet and syrup form, mainly for people who cannot manage inhalers; for example, the syrup can be useful for young children.

Although inhaled adrenaline-like drugs are very safe, they sometimes cause a fine tremor for a short time after inhalation. And if repeated dosages are necessary in quick succession, they may cause palpitations. The tablet and syrup forms have the same effect. **The tablet and syrup forms of reliever medication cannot be used repeatedly in an emergency situation like the inhaled reliever medication, as this could have dangerous side-effects. They are only to be used as prescribed by your doctor.**

THE REBOUND EFFECT

Potentially, there is a problem if the only medication you are taking is adrenaline-like reliever inhalers on a regular basis. If you use this type of medication about four times a day for more than two weeks, the airways get used to its actions. This has two effects. Firstly, the medication becomes less effective at relieving your asthma symptoms. Secondly, if you stop taking the medication, there may be rebound hyper-activity in your airways. If your airways are then exposed to an asthma trigger, a more marked asthma attack may occur that is difficult to treat. **You will be protected from this rebound effect by using regular preventative medication.** Also, ensure you do not run out of reliever medication by always having spares available.

ATROPINE-LIKE MEDICATION

This type of medication is derived from the plant *Atropa belladonna. Atropa* refers to its use as a poison, and *belladonna* to its once fashionable use by ladies to dilate their pupils. Examples of this medication are Atrovent (ipatropium) and Oxivent (oxitropium). These are not as effective as adrenaline-like reliever medication for treating asthma, but tend to be used for an older age group where they are useful for treating asthma in conjunction with bronchitis or emphysema. They are inhaled up to four times a day, and occasionally have the following side-effects: dry mouth, blurred vision and sometimes difficulty in passing water. Particular care needs to be taken if you suffer from the eye disease called glaucoma.

Add-on Medications

These medications are used in addition to the reliever and preventative medications already described. They are necessary under particular circumstances, such as wheezing at night or for asthma that is generally difficult to control.

XANTHINES

Examples of this type of medication are Nuelin (theo-phylline), Phyllocontin continus (aminophylline), Theo-dur or Uniphyllin continus. This type of medication acts like a reliever medication and may have some anti-inflammatory properties as well. It is important that its concentration in the bloodstream is neither too low, in which case it is not effective, nor too high, in which case side-effects, such as nausea or headaches, will be experienced. For this reason, regular blood tests will be necessary.

LONG-ACTING ADRENALINE-LIKE MEDICATION

These medications are similar to Bricanyl and Ventolin, except that their effects last a lot longer. Bricanyl and Ventolin will be effective for four to six hours, whereas the long-acting adrenaline-like medication will be effective for 12 hours. This medication is used in addition to preventative medication to achieve improved control of your asthma. There are two inhaled versions of this type of medication: Foradil (eformoteral fumarate), and Serevent (salmeterol). These medications are usually taken twice a day, regularly.

There are two important points to remember about Foradil and Serevent. Firstly, they *never* replace preventative medication. And secondly, they are not reliever medications. Although they will cause the airways to dilate like Ventolin or Bricanyl, they take a lot longer to do so. If you are using Foradil or Serevent, you will always have a preventative and reliever inhaler as well.

For people who find it difficult to use inhalers, there are two tablet preparations that are also taken twice a day, Bambec (bambuterol) and Volmax (salbutamol). The side-effects of the long-acting adrenaline-like medications are the same as for other adrenaline-like medications (see p. 40).

CORTICOSTEROID TABLETS

This type of medication is equivalent to steroid inhalers, except in tablet form. When there is quite a marked deterioration in a person's asthma these tablets deliver very high levels of steroids to the lungs in order to control the underlying inflammation. Steroid tablets are usually used in this way for three days to three weeks. **This is known as a short course of steroid tablets.** They may occasionally cause a tummy upset, water retention, mood swings and hyperactivity in children. However these side effects are not usually a problem.

Some very severe asthmatics are on **long-term** steroid tablets because this is the only way to control their asthma. Steroid side-effects can then be a problem, but usually only after many months or even years of continuous use. These side-effects include weight gain, thinning of the bones, thinning and bruising of the skin and raised blood pressure.

The generic name of the most commonly prescribed preparation is prednisolone. This comes as a small white or red tablet. The red tablet contains exactly the same medication as the white tablet except that it has a red sugar coating which makes it easier to swallow and also helps to prevent the stomach irritation that this medication sometimes causes. Pink, soluble tablets are available for children. Trade names for prednisolone in different markets are Prednesol (UK), Deltasolone (Aus) and Delta-Cortef (US and Canada).

If you are taking steroid tablets longterm, you must carry a steroid card, and only stop taking your steroids under medical supervision.

Inhalers

The purpose of asthma inhalers is to deliver medication deep into the lungs, to the sites of inflammation in the small and medium-sized airways. To get through to these airways the medication has to be in the form of very fine particles. Each inhalation contains vast numbers of medication particles so that they can be evenly spread throughout the equally vast number of small and medium-sized airways. Although there are many different inhalers available, they all fall into two main categories, *metered dose inhalers* and *dry powder inhalers*.

METERED DOSE INHALERS (MDIS)

This is the most common type of inhaler. The sealed metal canister sits inside a plastic holder. The metal canister contains the medication particles held in a mixture of chlorofluorocarbon (CFC) propellant. When you press the metal

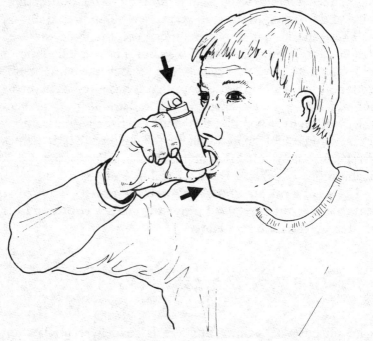

Using a metered dose inhaler (MDI)

THE CHLOROFLUOROCARBON (CFC) ISSUE

The Earth's ozone layer protects us from the damaging effects of ultra-violet rays from the sun. However the ozone layer itself is damaged by chlorofluorocarbons (CFCs), which are used as the propellant in MDIs and other aerosols, and in many industrial applications.

The 1981 Montreal Protocol requires all CFC production and use to be phased out by 1996, other than for essential purposes – as in MDIs.

A new propellant has now been developed called a hydrofluoroalkane (HFA), which is medically safe and ozone-friendly.

The first HFA (or CFC-free) inhalers were introduced in 1995. The first medication to be available with an HFA propellant was salbutamol. Preventative medication with the HFA propellant will be available in 1997 or 1998.

If you are prescribed an HFA inhaler you will notice a bitter taste when you take the medication. However the medication it delivers is exactly the same as that in your previous MDI.

It is possible that a small number of asthmatics will react unfavourably to the HFA propellant. If you are one of those people, you will notice a deterioration in your asthma five to ten minutes after using the MDI. If this is the case, inform your doctor immediately and do not use this MDI again.

canister down inside the plastic holder, the metering valve releases a precisely measured amount of propellant containing medication – a puff. The propellant drives the medication particles out of the MDI in the form of fast-moving droplets.

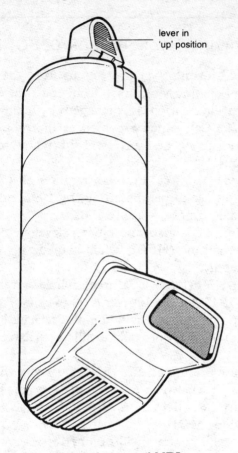

lever in
'up' position

A breath-actuated MDI

It is these droplets, containing both propellant and medication particles, that are inhaled.

About 50 per cent of asthma sufferers do not use MDIs correctly, which means they do not receive the correct medication. This is mainly because they find it difficult to coordinate pressing down the metal canister and breathing in at the same time.

However there are other ways of delivering asthma medication that do not require any coordination. If you use a

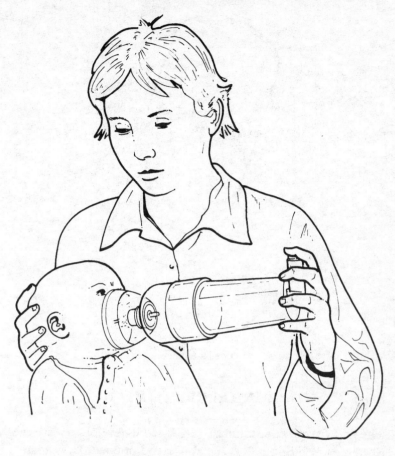

Using a spacer device with a mask attachment

breath-actuated MDI (see opposite), the inhaler is initially primed, and then automatically discharges as you breathe in. Alternatively, you can use a spacer device in which the MDI is discharged into the spacer, and you then breathe through the other end with normal breaths. For most people, a spacer is rather bulky to carry around, but it is particularly useful for small children and, with a mask attachment, for babies (see above).

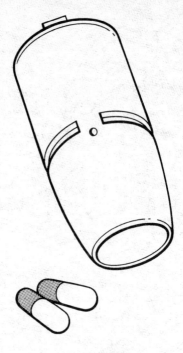

The Rotahaler

DRY POWDER INHALERS (DPIS)

The first dry powder inhalers (DPI) to be developed were the Rotahaler and Spinhaler (see above and opposite). A capsule containing a fine powder of medication particles held in lactose (a type of sugar) is inserted into the device. It is then primed by twisting the top sharply. You then put the DPI into your mouth and inhale, sucking the powder out (unlike an MDI which shoots out a fine spray). Priming the device and inhaling are two quite separate actions, not requiring any coordination. The lactose provides a characteristic sweet taste to let you know that you have taken the medication.

A number of DPIs, each with additional features, have been developed since the Rotahaler. The Diskhaler (see p. 50) has a disc containing either four or eight dosages of

48

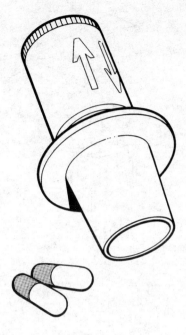

The Spinhaler

medication in separate blisters. The Turbohaler (see p. 50) has a reservoir containing enough medication for 50, 100, or 200 dosages. However it does not contain lactose and therefore has no taste. The Accuhaler (see p. 51) is a further development of the Diskhaler, containing 60 dosages in separate blisters.

There are many other asthma medications and delivery devices available but they all fall into one of the categories described. **If you have any doubts about the medication you have been prescribed, always ask your doctor or asthma nurse.**

Using the proper medication will enable you to lead your life free from the restraints that asthma may otherwise impose. In the next chapter we will see how to select the correct medication and the most appropriate delivery system so that you can be in control of asthma.

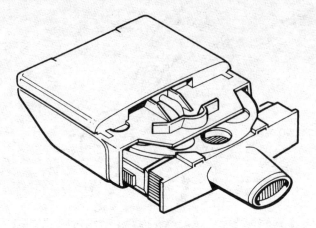

The Diskhaler

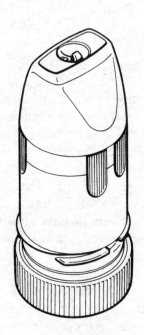

The Turbohaler

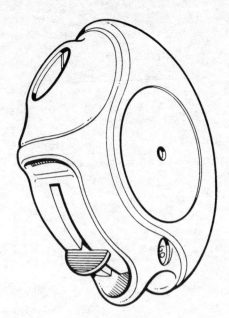

The Accuhaler

6

How To Be In Control Of Asthma

Uncontrolled asthma can impose major restrictions on your life, and is potentially life-threatening. However, by understanding the nature of asthma and the principles of asthma treatment, you can ensure your safety without restricting your lifestyle.

To recap, the main principles of asthma treatment are:

- Using preventative medication to control the inflammation in the airways.

- Prompt treatment of asthma symptoms using reliever medication.

- Taking simple commonsense measures to reduce your exposure to triggers as far as possible.

In partnership with your doctor or asthma nurse, you need to draw up an Asthma Management Plan to monitor your asthma and help you adjust your medication to meet changing demands. Asthma can be triggered by many factors, such as exercise or the house dust mite. Your personal management plan needs to include methods of dealing with changing circumstances as well as simple everyday measures you can take to reduce your exposure to triggers. It should also include a plan of action if you require urgent medical assistance.

No two management plans will be identical, but they all follow the same general principles. It is important that *your* Asthma Management Plan is tailored to meet *your own* needs, and ideally it should be written down. Your doctor should be able to provide a form for this purpose.

Monitoring Your Asthma

The first step towards being in control of your asthma is knowing the degree of inflammation present in your airways. The degree of inflammation is called your *asthma status*. If your asthma is under good control and there is no inflammation in your airways, then your asthma status is good. If your asthma has deteriorated and there is marked inflammation in your airways, then your asthma status is poor. You can assess your asthma status either *subjectively* (based on your own feelings), or *objectively* (based on external information) using a peak flow meter.

Some asthma sufferers can **subjectively** monitor their asthma status with great accuracy. These are *good monitors of asthma*. Other asthma sufferers' subjective monitoring of their asthma status is poor, so they are *poor monitors of asthma*. It is very important to know if you are a good or a poor monitor of asthma.

Good monitors experience symptoms with even minor changes in their asthma status and can therefore treat any deterioration straight away. Poor monitors may only experience asthma symptoms when there has already been a dangerous deterioration. People in this group are vulnerable to acute asthma attacks because of the delay in treating their deteriorating asthma status. Generally, if you have had acute asthma attacks previously, especially if any of them have resulted in a hospital admission, you are likely to be a poor monitor of asthma.

Poor monitors will only achieve good control of their asthma if they regularly use a peak flow meter to monitor their asthma status. The peak flow meter provides objective information, instead of relying on subjective feelings. Ideally, even good monitors of asthma should use a peak flow meter on a regular basis. Discuss this with your doctor or asthma nurse to decide whether a peak flow meter would be of benefit to you.

USING A PEAK FLOW METER TO MONITOR ASTHMA

Chapter 4 (pp. 28–31) describes how to use a peak flow meter and how it can be helpful in diagnosing asthma. The chart supplied with a peak flow meter is shown on p. 57. The first line to draw is line A, which represents your best peak flow reading. To work out where this line should be, you need to record your best peak flow readings on two or three days when you are completely well. **Remember, whenever you record a peak flow reading, it is the best reading out of three that is recorded.**

If your asthma is not well controlled when you first get your peak flow meter, you may need to have medication for some time before you can establish what your best peak flow readings are. Make sure you consult your doctor or asthma nurse when you draw line A, to ensure that your asthma is well controlled when you take these important readings, and that the line is correctly placed.

CALCULATING PERCENTAGES

This is very straightforward. For example, if your best peak flow reading is 500, and you wish to calculate 80

---

per cent of 500, all you have to do is multiply 500 by 0.8, e.g. $0.8 \times 500 = 400$.

If you wish to calculate 60 per cent of 500, all you have to do is multiply 500 by 0.6, e.g. $0.6 \times 500 = 300$.

Once line A has been drawn, two more lines can be added. These are the '80 per cent' and the '60 per cent' lines.

Your peak flow readings now fall into one of three bands:

- *Band 1* lies between line A and the 80 per cent line, and means that your asthma is well controlled and your medication does not need to be adjusted.

- *Band 2* lies between the 80 per cent line and the 60 per cent line. If your peak flow readings are in this band, this means that your asthma status has deteriorated, and you need to increase your medication. If you are already taking preventative medication, you probably need to double the amount you are taking. If you are not taking preventative medication, then you need to start doing so.

- *Band 3* lies below the 60 per cent line, and means that your asthma status has deteriorated to a dangerous level. In some Asthma Management Plans, this may mean you should start taking prednisolone tablets (see p. 43). In others it may mean that you should be using your reliever medication quite frequently to try and improve your asthma status, and you should be seeking urgent medical assistance. Your Asthma Management Plan should include details of how you will get urgent medical assistance if it becomes necessary.

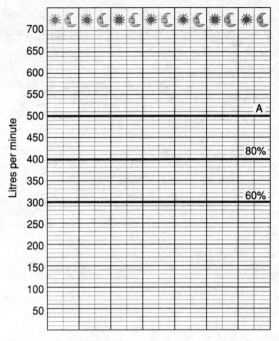

A peak flow chart showing a sample line A, and 80 per cent and 60 per cent lines

NORMAL PEAK FLOW CHARTS

Your peak flow meter will come with several charts to help you work out your expected peak flow according to your age, height and weight. However, there is a major problem with these charts because of the very wide range of readings they give. For example, according to these charts, a child who is 120 cm tall has a normal peak flow reading anywhere between 120 and 130 litres per minute. It is therefore more accurate to work out your own best peak flow reading, and leave it to your doctor or asthma nurse to ensure that it is what would be expected for a person of your age, sex and height.

The diagram below shows the peak flow chart of a well-controlled asthmatic. The peak flow readings are all in band 1, and form a fairly flat line.

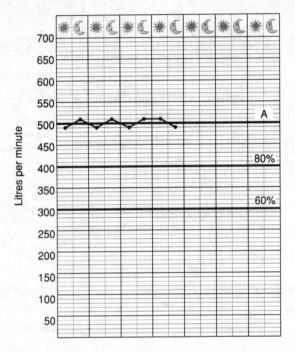

The peak flow chart of a well-controlled asthmatic

The chart opposite is that of a poorly-controlled asthmatic. Many of the peak flow recordings lie in band 2 and some even in band 3. This line is quite 'jagged' compared with the fairly flat line produced by the well-controlled asthmatic.

Once you have drawn line A, and the 80 per cent and 60 per cent lines, you can start to monitor your asthma status on a regular basis. The peak flow meter should be used twice a day, every day. The best times to use it are first thing in the morning and last thing at night. If you need to take reliever medication at either of these times, use the peak flow meter first.

The way you use your peak flow meter can be varied to suit your individual needs. Together with your doctor or asthma

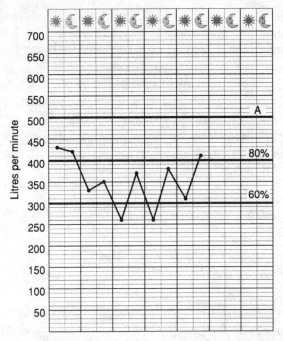

The peak flow chart of a poorly-controlled asthmatic

nurse, you may decide that the 80 per cent line should be a 70 per cent line, or that the 60 per cent line should be a 50 per cent line. Alternatively, after you have used the peak flow meter for some time, you may find that you are beginning to identify the early signs of deterioration in your asthma status, and then you can feel more confident about relying on your own subjective assessment. Then again, if your asthma is really quite unpredictable, it may be necessary to record your peak flow readings up to four times a day.

BRITTLE ASTHMA

Brittle asthma is a very unpredictable and severe form of asthma. The asthma sufferer can be entirely well, and then within a very short time find he is having a severe asthma attack. This can occur in spite of being on high doses of preventative medication.

Fortunately, this form of asthma is rare. Asthmatics with brittle asthma need to monitor their asthma status closely with a peak flow meter. In addition to working with their doctor and asthma nurse, people with brittle asthma should also have regular assessment and advice from a hospital specialist.

MONITORING ASTHMA WITHOUT A PEAK FLOW METER

Ideally, every asthmatic should monitor their asthma twice a day with a peak flow meter, but this may not fit in with your lifestyle. If you prefer to rely solely on your subjective assessment, it is a good idea to check first whether you are a good monitor of asthma. To do this, you need to start by working out your best peak flow measurement and drawing line A on the peak flow chart. Then calculate 85 per cent of your best value (0.85 × your best peak flow reading), and draw an 85 per cent line. Record your peak flow measurements four times a day, or at any time when you feel asthma symptoms, but *before* you use a reliever inhaler. Also, record on the chart any times when you felt breathless. If your peak flow falls below the 85 per cent line without you feeling asthma symptoms, then you are not a good monitor of asthma. See the peak flow chart shown opposite.

If you are a good monitor of asthma, you can monitor your asthma status and adjust your reliever medication according to the amount you need. Again, your peak flow readings will fall into one of three bands:

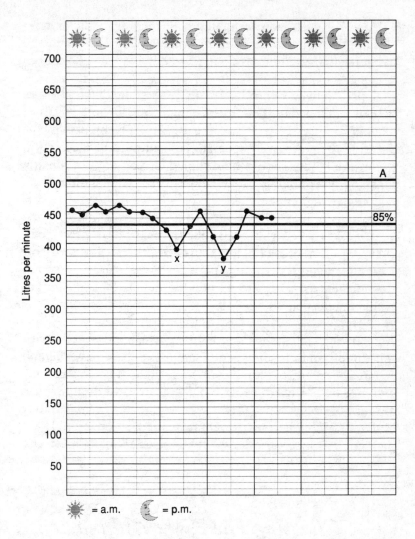

If you are aware of feeling breathless at, for example, points x and y, then you are a good monitor of asthma

- *Band 1* is when you are taking your reliever medication no more than once a day. This means that your asthma is well controlled, and there is no need to adjust your medication.

- *Band 2* is when you need your reliever medication more than once a day. This means that your asthma status is deteriorating. If you are already on preventative medication then, generally speaking, the amount of medication you are taking should be doubled. If you are not already taking preventative medication, then you should start doing so.

- *Band 3* is when you need reliever medication more than every four hours. **This is a dangerous situation and you need urgent medical attention.** Your Asthma Management Plan should include details of how you get this urgent help.

As you can see, these three bands correspond exactly with the three bands in the section on using peak flow meters. Again, the treatment can be varied in many ways to suit your own needs. For example, in band 2, instead of doubling the amount of preventative medication you take, you may find it better to increase your preventative medication by only 50 per cent. All such variations can be included in your Asthma Management Plan.

Choosing The Right Asthma Medication Delivery System

To be in control of your asthma you need to be sure that you are using the best delivery system for your asthma medication. Metered dose inhalers (MDIs) are the most commonly used delivery system, but only 50 per cent of people use MDIs correctly. This is because it can be quite difficult to coordinate pressing down the metal canister and breathing in at the same time. A simple way to tell if you are using your inhaler properly is to look in the mirror when you are taking a 'puff'. If you can see any of the medication escaping out of the corner of your mouth, this means you have not used the MDI correctly. If you have this problem with MDIs, discuss the situation with your doctor or asthma nurse. They may be able to help you use your MDI correctly, advise you to use your MDI with a spacer, or may encourage you to switch to either a dry powder device or a breath-actuated MDI. Elderly people with arthritic hands may find it helpful to use a Haleraid with their Ventolin (salbutamol) or Becotide (beclomethasone) MDIs, on sale at pharmacies. There is also the Turbohaler arthritis aid, available free from Astra Pharmaceuticals.

Some asthma sufferers do not like the taste of different types of inhalants. The CFC-free inhalants can taste quite bitter, and some of the dry powder devices can leave an unpleasant powdery sensation at the back of the mouth that some asthmatics find unpleasant. Turbohalers deliver only pure medication, and there is almost no taste or powdery sensation with this system.

MAKING SURE YOU NEVER RUN OUT OF MEDICATION IN AN MDI

Because asthma medication is concealed within a metal canister you cannot see how much medication is left. Although you can shake the canister and listen to the contents, this is not reliable. As we have seen, a major problem with taking adrenaline-like reliever inhalers on a regular basis is that if you suddenly stop taking them your asthma can get worse. This can happen if you run out of medication.

One way of checking how much medication is left in your MDI is to take the metal canister out of the plastic holder and place it in a bowl of water. If the canister sinks, it is full. If the canister floats, it is empty. In between is a matter of judgement. However this is a rather crude and inconvenient test, and some manufacturers advise against it, as it can cause damage to the MDI's valve mechanism.

The *only* way to make sure you do not run out of asthma medication is to **always be sure to have spare inhalers**.

The latest time for requesting spare inhalers, either preventative or reliever, is when you have just started your spare inhaler. However it is best if you request spare inhalers before this. In fact, it's a good idea to leave spare reliever inhalers in different places, for example in your car or in your office. If you find that you are still running out of asthma medication, you would probably be better off using a dry powder device such as an Accuhaler or a Turbohaler. The Accuhaler has a dose counter which shows how many doses have been used. In the Turbohaler a red indicator appears when 20 doses remain. This is the critical point at which to obtain a replacement inhaler.

CHOOSING THE RIGHT DELIVERY SYSTEM FOR BABIES AND CHILDREN

Most children under the age of about seven will not have the coordination to use an unmodified MDI. However an MDI with a spacer can be used by young children, and, with a mask attachment, even by babies. Using an MDI with a spacer does not require any coordination. Medication from the MDI is put in at one end, and the asthma sufferer takes normal breaths through the other end.

When children go to school they may find the spacer device too bulky to take with them. To overcome this problem, while they are still too young to use an unmodified MDI properly, a breath-actuated MDI can be used, such as an Autohaler, or a dry powder delivery system such as the Accuhaler or Turbohaler. As we have seen, none of these systems requires any coordination.

However, for babies and toddlers, even using a spacer together with an MDI may not prove to be satisfactory. This is because a certain amount of cooperation is still required to get a very young asthma sufferer to breathe through the spacer. Under these circumstances a nebuliser (shown on p. 66) may be useful. The mask is placed over the face and a fine mist is generated which contains the medication. The young asthma sufferer needs to wear the mask for about five minutes, breathing normally during this time.

However nebulisers do have drawbacks:

- They can make quite a lot of noise which upsets some children, although there is an almost silent nebuliser available.

- Also, parents may become over-reliant on the nebuliser, giving repeated dosages of reliever medication to treat a child's deteriorating asthma, rather than seeking medical assistance. If your child has a nebuliser take great care to discuss fully with your doctor or asthma nurse how it should, and should not, be used.

- Lastly, nebulisers cannot be prescribed by a doctor and are expensive to purchase. You may be lucky though – some surgeries have nebulisers which can be lent out. Make sure you return the nebuliser when you have finished with it because someone else will certainly need it.

Dealing With Triggers

If you are going to be exposed to a factor in the environment that you know triggers your asthma, you can either avoid the trigger, or eliminate it from the environment (for example, change bedding or remove pets). Alternatively, you can adjust your asthma medication to take into account your exposure to a known trigger.

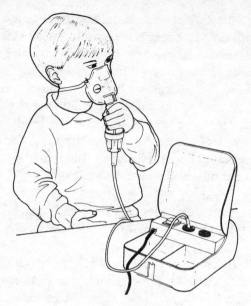

Using a nebuliser

CIGARETTE SMOKE

This is an example of a trigger that you may be able to largely avoid or eliminate from your environment. If you travel by train, always go in a no-smoking carriage. If guests who smoke come to your house, politely explain to them from the outset that, as a result of your asthma, you have a no-smoking policy in your house. Any considerate person will readily accept your request. If you are going to be in an environment where you cannot avoid being exposed to smoke (for example, in a pub), then take a dose of reliever medication before going there.

EXERCISE

This is a very common trigger of asthma, but not one to be avoided. Asthma sufferers can participate in any sport, pro-

66

viding their asthma is well controlled. If exercise triggers your asthma, take reliever medication about ten minutes before you start exercising and this will keep your asthma under good control. For children, an Intal inhaler (cromoglycate) used about half an hour beforehand is especially good for controlling exercise-induced asthma.

Skin Prick Testing

This is used to help to find out substances that you may be allergic to. A small sample of the substance is pricked beneath the skin using a needle. If there is redness and swelling some time later, this may mean that you are allergic to the substance. This test is not particularly reliable and, as there can be a severe reaction, it is only available at specialist centres.

THE HOUSE DUST MITE

While it may not be possible to eliminate house dust mites from your house altogether, it is possible to keep them to a minimum by taking a number of cheap and simple measures such as:

- damp dusting;

- using vinyl flooring or tiles instead of carpets where possible;

- covering mattresses, pillows and duvets with allergen-proof casings (available from large stores);

- and regular vacuuming.

If you suffer from asthma and you can possibly get someone else to do the vacuuming for you, then you should do so. This is because, although vacuuming reduces the house dust mite population, it actually throws mite faeces into the air, possibly making asthma worse. If you have to vacuum yourself, make sure you use a vacuum cleaner with a good filter, and a paper collection bag rather than a cloth one which allows small particles through. You could also wear a mask (available from your pharmacy).

DIET

Certain foods, and many food additives, have been found to exacerbate asthma in a small number of cases. The difficulty in deciding whether you are reacting to a food or food additive is that the reaction may come on many hours afterwards. Keeping a diary and noting when you have eaten a suspect food and when you have experienced an exacerbation of your asthma may help to clarify the matter. If the situation is still

---

THE EXCLUSION DIET

To begin with, you need to eliminate almost all foods apart from one or two basics which are known to be virtually free from triggers. Lamb and pears are examples of such foods. Regular peak flow meter readings are taken for a few days before the diet begins, and then during it. One by one, regular foods are re-introduced to the diet. If one item is the trigger, the peak flow readings will deteriorate after a day or two. The whole process must then be repeated to ensure that the poor peak flow reading was not due to an entirely different trigger.

---

unclear, you could try an exclusion diet. **As an exclusion diet involves a major change to your diet for some time, you must be under the supervision of your doctor.**

Review Appointments

It is important for your Asthma Management Plan to include regular review appointments with your doctor or asthma nurse, usually about once every three months, or more frequently if your asthma is not well controlled. On these occasions you can review your asthma status over the previous three months and make any changes that are necessary. For instance, you may wish to change your medication delivery system, adjust the amount of preventative treatment you are taking, or discuss how best to deal with any particularly troublesome circumstances.

You can have good control of your asthma provided:

- you are well informed about asthma;

- you have a 'partnership' with your doctor or asthma nurse;

- careful consideration is given to your particular needs.

Dr Mark Britton is a hospital-based chest specialist who looks after those asthmatic patients whose condition is so serious or difficult to control that either their doctor has referred them to him, or they have been admitted to the hospital with acute asthma attacks.

'My aim', says Dr Britton, is to treat patients so that they are well, do any exercise they want to and go on to take a full part in life.'

Initially he reassures his asthma patients that no matter how uncontrolled their asthma is now, with the correct medication and with proper care and attention to detail the quality of their lives should be significantly improved. At the same time he makes sure that they understand the seriousness of their condition.

He treats patients from the age of five upwards, and is as likely to see a 60-year-old as a 16-year-old. 'There is no "asthma personality",' he says. 'I do not believe that "nerves" cause asthma – but it is a frightening illness, and the fear can influence the child's emotional development and give rise to a nervous personality. However that is brought about by the asthma, it does not bring the asthma about.'

There was a time when many patients who were referred to Dr Britton had been prescribed the correct medication but were having problems because they did not know how to take their medication correctly, or else had forgotten. However since asthma nurses have become a part of many health centres, patient compliance and inhaler techniques are much improved.

Many of Dr Britton's patients come because their asthma has suddenly worsened and become out of control. This is often due to a viral infection like a heavy cold thwarting the anti-inflammatory action of the asthma medication. He believes that many patients can be taught to adjust their medication to take account of this.

There is a small group of patients whose asthma is difficult to keep stable. These are the patients with **brittle asthma**. Their type of asthma is sudden and unpredictable, and a severe attack can occur for no apparent reason. 'I alert them to the severity of their problem, and the need for great care,' says Dr Britton. 'Together we work out strategies for dealing with brittle asthma emergencies. To be most effective this has to involve the whole family.'

So why has there been such a huge increase in the number of asthmatics? Dr Britton believes that nowadays diagnosis is more accurate. Previously, smokers with chest problems were diagnosed as having smoking-related bronchitis. Now with the percentage of smokers in the population being far less, chest problems are increasingly being recognised as asthma.

Dr Britton is forthright in his approach to asthma diagnosis and treatment. 'In my definition cough, wheeze and shortness of breath equals asthma,' he says. 'It is the diameter of the small airways that brings about the symptoms: a minute change in the diameter of an infant's airways has a dramatic effect on the airflow in the lungs. As the child grows and his airways get proportionately wider, the narrowing caused by inflammation may have less of an effect on his breathing, and his asthma may seem to abate. Inhaled steroids should be used to treat asthma as soon as it is diagnosed: a chronic inflammatory condition in the lungs that rumbles on untreated can lead to damage of the airways, and chronic problems in later life. People never fully "grow out" of asthma, the potential is always there for it to return.'

Dr Mark G. Britton is Consultant Physician and Medical Director at St Peter's Hospital NHS Trust, Chertsey, Surrey.

Although this chapter gives general advice about adjusting asthma medication, you must *only* self-adjust medication according to the Asthma Management Plan agreed with your doctor or Asthma nurse.

7

How To Cope In An Emergency

'If only I had realised how bad it was . . .'
'If only I had known that people die from asthma . . .'

Effective asthma treatment aims to eliminate the 'if only', by
giving asthma sufferers and those around them the *knowledge*
to realise when a situation is life-threatening, and the *confidence* to take emergency action promptly.

How To Recognise An Acute Asthma Attack

When inflammation in the airways interferes with the movement of air in and out of the lungs, the asthma sufferer
experiences symptoms such as wheezing, coughing and
recession (drawing in of the flesh between the ribs and above
the sternum). In an acute asthma attack these symptoms
become more marked, or may even change in nature. The
asthmatic often becomes quiet and withdrawn, concentrating
on the fight for breath. He will typically sit in the position
shown in the diagram below. This enables him to brace the
muscles of his upper body and helps him expand his chest, in

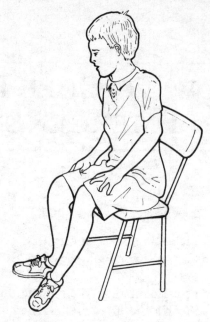

A child displaying the features of an acute asthma attack

opposition to the huge resistance in his lungs. The long expiratory wheeze at first becomes louder, and the short inspiratory gulp may become quite harsh. The recession will become more marked.

If you have a peak flow meter, generally a reading 50 per cent below your best peak flow reading (line A, see page 59) indicates that you are having an acute asthma attack. However you may not be able to use a peak flow meter if your asthma has already reached a critical stage.

As the situation continues to deteriorate, the airways become more inflamed and the movement of air slows even further. At this point, there is so little air movement in and out of the lungs that the expiratory wheeze and harsh inspiratory gulp are no longer audible. There is even insufficient air movement for the asthmatic to say more than one or two words, or perhaps none at all. Many asthmatics have died because of this situation. The wheeze and the inspiratory gulp have disappeared; the asthmatic is quiet and withdrawn. Under these circumstances, parents, teachers, spouses, friends and even doctors have all mistakenly assumed that the asthmatic is improving, failed to take the appropriate course of action, and the result has been another avoidable asthma death.

A desperately urgent situation has arrived when:

• The asthmatic is unable to say more than one or two words (if any).

• There is marked recession (drawing in of the flesh between the ribs and above the sternum). Recession is a useful sign of acute asthma because it tends to become more marked as the situation deteriorates – unlike the wheeze and the harsh inspiratory gulp which, paradoxically, can appear to improve as an acute attack worsens. **But beware: an asthmatic can have a severe asthma attack without marked recession.**

• An additional feature, called cyanosis, may develop. This is when the lips and tongue turn grey/blue because there is so little oxygen in the blood. This can be a difficult feature to recognise but, once present, death can quickly follow unless the person receives professional medical help.

At this critical stage, an asthmatic will find using a peak flow meter extremely difficult. If he is reluctant to use the peak flow meter don't force the issue – trying to use a peak flow meter under these circumstances can actually make asthma worse. Under these circumstances you will have to judge the severity of the attack by how the asthmatic appears.

Who Develops An Acute Asthma Attack?

Perhaps surprisingly, the people most likely to suffer acute asthma attacks are those who have had a number of attacks before. These people are inclined not to notice that their condition is worsening because the special monitoring receptors in their lungs fail to alert them to changes brought about by the increasing inflammation. Unfortunately, they fail to notice their deteriorating lung function until the asthma attack is critical.

Many of those who suffer acute asthma attacks are people who fail to take their preventative medication. Rachel is a typical example.

Sixteen-year-old Rachel went on holiday with a group of friends to the Devon coast. She had not bothered to pack her Pulmicort (budesonide) and so had been without any preventative inhaler for five days. On the last night she went to an all-night beach barbecue, where she sat around a smoky bonfire, sang, laughed, ran in the sea and became thoroughly chilled.

Around 4 am, as she shivered near the dying embers of the fire, her chest began to tighten. She had no reliever inhaler, and was too embarrassed to ask if any of the other partygoers had one. By sunrise Rachel was in an acute asthmatic state, and had to be taken to hospital. She recovered this time – luckily!

Also vulnerable to acute attacks are those people who have obediently followed the advice of their doctor, when unfortunately their doctor has failed to prescribe preventative medication, or has prescribed an insufficient dosage. It is thought that about half of all asthmatics are not adequately treated.

It must be stressed that *anyone* can have a sudden asthma attack, even people who have never had asthma, or symptoms of asthma, before. One of the hallmarks of asthma is its unpredictability. This first attack can be fatal in less than one hour, unless professional medical help is sought.

When Is An Acute Asthma Attack Likely To Occur?

The most likely time for a severe attack to occur is during the night or early morning. Most asthmatics say that their asthma is at its worst at these times. There are thought to be two reasons for this. As we have seen, the most potent household trigger is the house dust mite, and this little creature particularly favours the bedroom. However the influence of the body's natural rhythms is probably of greater significance.

Because of these rhythms we produce lower levels of the hormones adrenaline and cortisone, a natural steroid, during our sleep. Both these substances are chemical messengers which act as the body's natural anti-asthma medications. As they lessen during the night, the likelihood of an asthma attack increases.

However, an acute asthma attack can develop at any time, day or night, especially if asthmatics are exposed to triggers such as cold air, animal dander, cigarette smoke or viral infections.

How To Manage Acute Asthma

There are a number of conditions, such as hyperventilation, that even experienced doctors find difficult to distinguish from asthma. So the golden rule, if you suspect that a person may be having an acute asthma attack, is *always* to treat them for an acute asthma attack. Even if they have never had asthma before, their first attack could be acute. So the safest option is to give them the appropriate treatment for acute asthma. Even if they turn out not to have asthma, you won't have done any harm.

These are the steps you should take to deal with such a crisis effectively:

- Do not panic. Asthma worsens in an atmosphere of panic. So, although you are bound to feel panicky, this feeling must not be transmitted to the asthmatic. He is to some extent out of control, and is best helped by feeling that those around him are in control.

- Give the asthmatic a means of raising the alarm in the middle of the night. This could be as simple as keeping a noisy school bell at the bedside – as long as the bell is light enough to be lifted and rung effectively. Or it could be as complicated as installing an electric alarm. It could indeed be any device that does not rely on the asthmatic having to shout or exert himself, because he will be unable to do so.

- Give inhaled reliever medication, such as Bricanyl (terbutaline) or Ventolin (salbutamol). There may be a good response from a single dose, in which case the urgency is lessened. From then on the important action is to observe that the attack does not begin again. If it does, give more reliever medication.

- If you have a peak flow meter, it can be useful to judge if the asthma attack is getting better or worse. It is particularly useful for judging if there has been improvement after using reliever medication.

- If there is no response to a single dose, give more inhaled reliever medication. In an emergency situation it may be necessary to give an asthmatic 40 doses or more of reliever medication from a metered dose inhaler or dry powder inhaler.

- If the asthmatic does not have his own reliever medication at hand, use someone else's. This is quite acceptable in a situation which is, or may become, an emergency.

- As the asthma attack develops, breathing in (inspiration) will become so difficult that the asthmatic will not be able to use his inhalers in the normal way. In these circumstances, a nebuliser or a spacer can be very useful, as they do not require any inspiratory effort. With the nebuliser, the asthmatic breathes through the mask; and, with the spacer, he breathes through the mouthpiece. For emergency purposes a makeshift spacer can be improvised (see diagram below), using a plastic cup with a hole in one end, a cut-up plastic bottle or even a cup made from tin foil. The wide end is placed over the mouth, and the inhaler is puffed repeatedly into the hole at the other end. The asthmatic breathes 'normally' and takes in the reliever medication without further exertion.

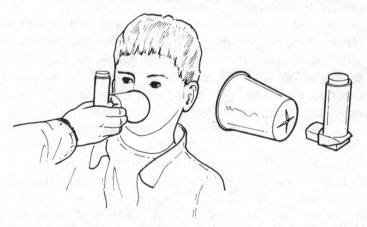

In an emergency, you can use a paper cup as a makeshift spacer

Knowing when and how to seek professional medical help can pose a problem for those around an asthma sufferer. If any feature of an acute asthma attack is present, and particularly if it persists despite using reliever medication, professional medical help is urgently needed.

Remember, 25 per cent of deaths from asthma happen within one hour of the onset of an acute asthma attack.

How you obtain professional medical help will depend on where you live and the quality of the services available. The usual course of action is to contact your doctor. An asthma-aware doctor will quickly assess the severity of the attack by asking one or two pertinent questions. He may then choose to make a home visit (if this service is provided), to examine the asthmatic in the surgery, or to advise you to go straight to casualty. Unfortunately not all doctors are as asthma-aware as they might be. In about one-third of asthma deaths, studies have shown that the doctor did not accurately assess the severity of the final attack, and thus failed to take the appropriate course of action.

If you are not entirely satisfied with the service your doctor is providing – perhaps he is unable to visit, maybe you are unable to get past the receptionist – then take control of the situation and find help elsewhere.

If you are near a hospital with a casualty department, go straight there. A person with a severe asthma attack needs oxygen and nebulised reliever medication. If you are without transport, then dial 999 and call an ambulance. All ambulances are now equipped with oxygen and nebulisers, and ambulance crews are trained to deal with asthma attacks. If you live in a rural area a long way from the nearest hospital, it is best to dial 999 and follow the advice of the ambulance control: there may be an ambulance nearby.

Once you arrive in a casualty department, the situation is not necessarily plain sailing. In the reception area, you have to impress upon the clerical staff the severity of the problem in order to gain quick access to the medical staff. Even if

'When my son had his first severe asthma attack I thought at first that he was actually getting better. Instead of wheezing and coughing he had quietened down, and seemed to be calm. It was not until we realised he could barely speak to us that we began to panic. We rang 999, and I remember shouting "BAD ASTHMA ATTACK" down the telephone – but it worked. The ambulance arrived within minutes and my son was given oxygen immediately.

He made a complete recovery in hospital.

The trouble is though, I'm frightened. Suppose it happens again? What else can I do to help him?'

people in the waiting area appear to have far more dramatic problems than your asthma sufferer, you are going to have to jump the queue. So **be pushy, be firm**. The words that will activate the alarm are simple, 'SEVERE ASTHMA ATTACK.' If they are said with conviction they will get a response even from the meanest of hospital receptionists.

The casualty doctor will assess the patient who, if necessary, will be given oxygen and concentrated reliever medication via a nebuliser. If there is not a satisfactory response, he will then be given reliever medication and steroids, such as cortisone, via an intravenous drip, in a further attempt to open up the airways. He should respond fairly quickly to this treatment and be breathing more easily in quite a short while. If intravenous treatment is required, the asthmatic will almost certainly be admitted to the ward for a day or two. This is usually taken as a good opportunity to adjust his medication. If you have been to casualty or admitted to hospital for asthma, it is important to see your own doctor or asthma nurse to review your Asthma Management Plan.

Never worry that you may be bothering the doctor or the hospital unnecessarily. Doctors understand and deal with genuine medical problems: it is part of their job. And the person in your house with an acute asthma attack has a major medical problem that must be dealt with – immediately.

There is an important hidden danger in the system, whether it is the doctor or hospital that treats the acute asthma attack. An acute asthmatic will typically be given nebulised reliever medication. Often this dramatically improves the situation, and the asthmatic goes home. However, as we have already seen, asthma is caused by inflammation in the airways, and this inflammation can take many days to settle. Even if there has been a quick recovery after minimal treatment, it is always vital to observe an asthmatic with great care, especially in the period just after an acute asthma attack.

Peter's asthma had been bad and so at 4 pm his mother took him to see his doctor. He was treated with a nebuliser and seemed to respond well. Confident that, as he had seen the doctor and had been nebulised, he must be better, his mother took him home. He seemed quiet and tired, and as he had had a disturbed night previously she put him to bed. But Peter's attack was merely temporarily relieved by the medication, not cured and his condition deteriorated rapidly in the night. Fortunately his mother kept a close watch on him and was able to act swiftly to prevent a fatality.

If you have needed nebulised reliever medication to relieve your asthma attack, then you will also need a course of oral steroid tablets to treat the ongoing inflammation. If you do not have your own supply of steroid tablets, and instructions on how to use them in your Asthma Management Plan, consult your own doctor soon.

Around 2,000 people die of asthma each year, and nearly all these deaths are preventable. One of the most dangerous scenarios is when an attack occurs suddenly in a person who is not known to be asthmatic. Not surprisingly, people are slow to react to this situation, and the delay can prove fatal.

Another particularly dangerous scenario is when a doctor fails to assess the severity of an attack. Doctors are fallible. So if your instinct says that the situation is more serious than the doctor says, listen to that instinct and go to hospital.

It cannot be emphasised enough that anyone with a severe asthma attack is safest in hospital. So **if in doubt, go to casualty**.

8

HOW WILL ASTHMA AFFECT YOUR LIFE?

Being asthmatic can sometimes feel like being at odds with the world. Certainly, once asthma comes into your life, you will need to make allowances for it and perhaps even change some of your priorities. **However, as long as your asthma is properly managed, life can go on pretty much as normal.**

> *The worst of my asthma attack is over and I feel almost right, though now and again I resort to my new acquisition, a French inhaler . . .*
> from 'The Motorcycle Diaries', *A Journey Around South America,* Verso 1995

Who would have thought that these words had been written in 1952 by Che Guevara, the Latin American revolutionary? Whatever your politics, you would probably agree that Che did not allow his asthma to prevent him from making his mark in the world!

There is no need to feel that having asthma will stop you leading a full life, that because your child has asthma he will fail to become the athlete, footballer or rounded personality he might have been, or that your elderly asthmatic relative should forego shopping trips and outings in case of an asthma attack.

Whether you suffer from asthma yourself or you are caring for someone who does, there are three important points to bear in mind:

• You will need to be aware of your **immediate environment**. Once you have established what triggers your asthma, you may be able to conveniently avoid some of those triggers, using simple commonsense measures.

• You will need to be **vigilant when caring for asthma sufferers**. They don't always realise or effectively communicate how serious their asthma is.

• You will need to **take care of yourself**. It is particularly important for asthma sufferers to look after their general health.

Coping With Asthma At Home

INDOORS

Dust mites can be kept down with regular vacuuming and dusting, and removed from clothing, bedding and towels through very hot washing. Animal dander can be eliminated or at least kept to certain rooms. Don't forget soft toys; they too need regular washing and airing. Carpets and rugs need vacuuming and shaking, but be aware of the danger of flying dust when shaking out rugs, blankets or curtains. At the very least, you should do this outdoors. Better still, ask a non-asthmatic to take the items outside and give them a good shake.

If you are allergic to the pollen of heavily scented flowers, they should not be brought into the house.

Sealed and double-glazed windows inhibit the flow of fresh air in the home. Our grandparents urged us to throw open the windows each morning because 'fresh air does you good'.

They were right – it does. Asthmatics are sensitive to the state of the air, and stale, dusty or smoky air in the home bothers them. (However, do remember that 'fresh' air can also trigger asthma if it contains high quantities of pollen, pollution, or even just because it is cold.)

If you are asthmatic, doing the housework can provoke an attack due to the disturbance of dust. To alleviate this problem, many asthmatics wear a simple facial dust mask when doing dusty jobs. These are inexpensive and can be bought from high street chemists. Creosote and other anti-woodworm compounds, fresh paint and any chemicals should also be avoided.

OUTDOORS

Gardens are teeming with asthma triggers: seasonal grass pollen and tree pollen, moulds and spores released from fungi, smoke, dust, cold air, and so on. However, some of these triggers can be minimised. For example, by not having bonfires (and by educating your neighbours into not having them) you will be giving yourself cleaner air to breathe.

Gardens can even be designed to include plants that are kind to asthma sufferers; this is called *low allergen gardening*. Most trees (except fruit trees), grasses and wild flowers are wind-pollinated, and so release their pollen into the air. This pollen is a major asthma trigger. In a low allergen garden you would avoid these plants in favour of insect-pollinated plants such as herbs, most shrubs (except the heavily scented ones like jasmine and honeysuckle), most low-scented flowers, water plants and fruit trees. As mowing can trigger asthma, lawns should be avoided and perhaps be replaced with terraces and tubs. Hedges, too, spell danger for asthmatics since they can trap dust and pollen from other plants which are released into the air when the hedges are trimmed.

ENTERTAINING

Asthma can also affect your social life at home. For example, a dinner party should be a relaxed fun evening of indulgence in food, wine and good company. But what if there is a heavy smoker among the guests? What if you are allergic to the shellfish? What if the strain of preparing dinner for ten people *and* trying to get the children into bed is all too much for you? And what if the evening is such a success that you become helpless with laughter? All these factors can trigger asthma.

However, with some thought and effort, the risks can be diminished. Your immediate environment can be improved simply by banning smoking in your house. If your guest is that desperate for a cigarette, he will just have to smoke outside. When planning the menu, you can make sure that you avoid all foods to which you know you are allergic, and err on the side of caution when you are unsure.

Slotting ten or fifteen minutes into the schedule in which to lie down and relax will ease the pressure and keep you calm. If this means that you have to offer a less ambitious meal, or that the children have to miss out on their bedtime story that night, so be it. And if the laughter around the table is uncontrollable, a puff of your reliever inhaler will help your airways to cope.

SEX

There are other important areas in which asthma may affect your life at home. Sex can trigger a form of exercise-induced asthma. You might take a puff of reliever before an energetic aerobics class: you could do the same before sex. Since some asthmatics experience a feeling of panic if heavy pressure is applied to their chests, you may have to rethink your positioning. You should certainly never experiment with any form of artificial restraint around the chest if asthmatic.

PREGNANCY

The most important point about asthma and pregnancy is that uncontrolled asthma can be dangerous for the unborn child. This is because, when you are having a serious asthma attack, your body is receiving lower than normal levels of oxygen. Since the baby obtains its oxygen directly from the mother's supply, it too will be deprived of this life-giving substance.

In order to avoid asthma affecting their lives at such an important time, pregnant women must take care of themselves. This means keeping up your regular medication, and seeing your doctor promptly if your asthma is showing any sign of getting out of control. He may prescribe other drugs, such as antibiotics for a chest infection. Though you may prefer to avoid such medication during pregnancy, if you have a bad attack of asthma because you have not taken the medication prescribed for you, then you are putting your baby's well-being at risk. If you do need an antibiotic, your doctor will choose one that does not harm your baby.

Some women find that their asthma improves during pregnancy. This is because the same hormones that prevent rejection of the placenta also reduce inflammation in the airways. However others find that their asthma worsens. This may be due to stress or simply to their increasingly large abdomen reducing the space available for their lungs, causing shortness of breath.

Before the actual birth, the midwife, doctor and nurses should all be informed that you are asthmatic, in case you need a general anaesthetic. This is because, if you have an acute asthma attack while under general anaesthetic, your lung function may deteriorate. The anaesthetist needs to know quickly what is causing this to happen, so that he can give the correct drugs. This applies to any operation requiring an anaesthetic.

BREASTFEEDING

Inhaled asthma medication does not get into breast milk in sufficient quantities to affect the baby, and indeed there is some evidence to say that breastfeeding protects the baby against allergies. If your baby has inherited your atopic tendency (see p. 175), this will be in his genes already. He will not acquire such a tendency through breastfeeding.

FIGHTING BACK

Whatever measures you take at home, you may sometimes feel as if asthma is running your life. One way of handling this is to fight back. Asthma affects Catherine's life, but she takes control.

Catherine's asthma is triggered by cigarette smoke. Her friends know this and would never smoke in her presence. She avoids pubs, always asks for a non-smoking table in restaurants and has even been upgraded on an aeroplane because there were no seats left in the non-smoking area. She refuses to run the risk of an asthma attack simply because she was too weak-willed to assert her need for clean air.

This is precisely how the mothers of children in Greenwich, South London, coped with the increase in asthma among children living around Trafalgar Road, an area notorious for traffic pollution. In times of extremely poor air quality, these mothers believed the road ought to be closed, as the weight of traffic was worsening the air pollution and thus, they felt, triggering bad attacks in their asthmatic children. They fought back by trying to force the council into implementing such road closures when the need arose.

Fighting back could involve joining a pressure group campaigning for cleaner air, less traffic or more asthma awareness in schools.

Coping With Asthma Away From Home

You mentioned your name as if I should recognise it, but beyond the obvious facts that you are a bachelor, a solicitor, a Freemason, and an asthmatic, I know nothing whatever about you . . .

from *The Memoirs of Sherlock Holmes* by Sir Arthur Conan Doyle

Thankfully asthma treatment has moved on significantly since Sherlock Holmes' time, and nowadays the disease need not be an *obvious problem*. Indeed an asthma sufferer may well surprise his friends when he mentions that he is asthmatic.

SPORT

Many sportsmen and sportswomen achieve their full potential, despite being asthmatic. Here are a few inspiring examples.

Adrian Moorhouse MBE
Adrian Moorhouse was an asthmatic boy who took up swimming because the people around him said that he ought to get fit in order to get better, and because swimming was the only sport he could do. 'I wanted to be healthy, I needed to find a way to escape from my asthma,' he says – and he went on to become a world champion.

His achievements include ranking first in the world for

100 metres breaststroke for five years, winning the Olympic gold medal, four European Gold Medals and three Commonwealth Games Gold Medals, swimming in every major competition from 1981 to 1992 (including three Olympic Games), and becoming the first man ever to break one minute for the 100m breast stroke short course.

Adrian Moorhouse's asthma has usually been triggered by a cold or bronchitis. He remembers broken nights during his childhood, propped up against piles of pillows, tight-chested and wheezy. 'Although I was never admitted to hospital with an asthma attack, there were times when I probably should have been,' he says.

He was prescribed Ventolin tablets, and during the winter was given allergy tests and courses of 'desensitising' injections. Around the age of eight the asthma specialist gave him some advice which stayed with him and which probably led him to fulfil his sporting potential and become a world champion athlete.

The advice was:

- Carry on swimming, take it to your own limit and don't let anyone else put limitations on you.

- Let the people around you know that you are asthmatic, so that they can take action if you get into difficulties.

Armed with this advice, he swam regularly, became fitter and 'told my teacher to pull me out if I start struggling'. By the age of eleven he was exercising, swimming and working out eight times a week. He was also taking Intal, via a Spinhaler, to treat his asthma.

During his early teens his asthma was under control most of the time, although there were occasions when he had to pull out of competitions. This usually happened when he had a cold which went to his chest. If he did not rest, the cold would turn to bronchitis and trigger his asthma. He now needed occasional Ventolin as well as Intal.

At the age of fourteen Adrian Moorhouse moved to a new swimming club, took up weight training, grew a lot and became stronger. The following year he joined the England International Team as a junior and, later that year, as a senior. Then he went on to conquer the world.

Adrian Moorhouse has learnt to manage his asthma. It has always been at its worst during October, November and December, so when success came he managed to escape the British winter by spending those months in the warm climates of America or Australia. This enabled him to train hard and reach a peak of fitness in time for the European competitions in January.

Since retiring from competitive swimming in 1992 he has founded a successful management consultancy. He works out in the gym and remains involved with swimming via charities, clubs and the media.

He is firmly of the opinion that the advice which he was given as a boy (Don't let anyone limit you but let them know you are asthmatic) could well be given to any asthmatic child who felt that the condition was dominating their life.

Karen MacLeod

As a child growing up on the Isle of Skye, Scotland, Karen MacLeod developed hayfever. Her mother and sister had it too, and Karen's condition was bad enough to require strong anti-histamine tablets to dampen down the symptoms. She still has memories of feeling sluggish in class, due to the effect of these tablets.

Then she moved to Bath, England, and her hayfever worsened. Meanwhile she was re-kindling her childhood enthusiasm for running. She began to enter 'fun-runs' and short road races. But springtime became the season of misery. She battled with breathing problems which began as soon as pollens were dispersed into the air, and during that pollen time exercise seemed to add to her difficulties.

By 1984 the hobby had become a passion, and Karen was selected to run for Scotland.

The following year Karen's doctor diagnosed her as asthmatic, but she was unwilling to accept his diagnosis. She also disliked the Ventolin she was given as it 'gave me the shakes and made my heart race'. Later she was prescribed Intal, which seems to control her allergic asthma. She takes it from mid-March until late August. Her normal dosage is two or three times a day, although she will increase this before a strenuous session on the track.

Since 1984 she has represented Scotland in four world championship cross country races, and was a member of the Scottish team for the 1990 Commonwealth Games in New Zealand, where she ran the 10,000 metres.

Karen has also run for Great Britain, notably the marathon in the 1993 World Championships Track and Field in Stuttgart, and in the 1994 Commonwealth Games in Canada. She hopes to run the marathon again for Great Britain in the 1996 Olympics in Atlanta.

Karen's strength is in her endurance, which is why she has concentrated on marathon running for the past few years. However, she has had to face up to the fact that for a few months of the year she has asthma attacks. 'The attacks are predictable,' she says. 'I run on a disused railway line between Bath and Bristol, which is bordered by trees and high grassy banks. One day in March or April I can run down there comfortably, the next day I'm suffocating, there is so much dust and pollen in the air.'

Karen is well aware that her kind of exercise exacerbates her asthma. Running miles across countryside, through fields or on recently mown tracks, coupled with the amount of air that is passing in and out of her lungs during this extremely strenuous exercise is bound to bring problems, especially during the pollen season.

Karen's schedule for a typical weeks' training is as follows:

	morning	*afternoon*
Sunday	long run of 22 miles	4 miles 'easy' to ease legs
Monday	5 miles easy road running	5 miles easy
Tuesday	on the track, 20 × 400 m, with a 100 m recovery jog between each 400 m. 3 miles warm up and warm down	4 miles on road
Wednesday	short 5 mile run	15–18 mile run
Thursday	on the track, about 10 × 1,000 m, with a 200 m recovery jog between each, and a 3 mile warm up or down	5 miles easy, plus stretching
Friday	'rest day', perhaps just a five mile gentle run	
Saturday	on the track, interval sessions of various distances from 200 m to 2 miles at a fast pace	4 miles easy, plus stretching

Karen sticks to this schedule when in training, treating her asthma with Intal. Without this medication there would be times when she simply could not run. On a dry, windy day in April she is likely to become breathless and wheezy. 'I have only ever had real problems with my asthma when I have been putting my body under stress', she says. 'Hurtling round the track inhaling all those allergens can trigger my asthma. Then I am unable to regain composure between efforts, my breathing becomes harder and more laboured. Sometimes in panic I have hyperventilated.'

'Although I have rebelled in the past and denied that I was asthmatic, I know that there are certain times every year when I have to take asthma medication.

Asthma is undoubtedly a frightening disease, but it need not restrict your life if you watch out for it and treat it properly.'

Steve Ovett

Steve Ovett broke the world record three times for running 1500 metres, twice for running the mile and once for running two miles. He won the Olympic Gold in 1980 for the 800 metres, the IAAF Gold Cup in 1977 and 1981 for the 1500 metres, and was European Champion for the 1500 metres in 1978. He is asthmatic.

Alan Pascoe MBE

Between 1966 and 1978 Alan Pascoe represented the British Athletics Team in five different events. As well as captaining the British team, he won Gold in the 400 metre hurdles in the Commonwealth Games, and two double Golds in the European Championships. He also won the European Indoor Championships, two European Cup finals and gained an Olympic Silver medal at the Munich Games.

In 1975 he was ranked Number One in the world for the 400 metre hurdles and was also awarded an MBE for his services to sport.

Alan Pascoe is asthmatic.

Of course we won't all go on to become world-class athletes, whether or not we have asthma. But the important point is that if an asthma sufferer *does* want to take part in any sport there is no reason for asthma to prevent such activity. Taking exercise is an important part of looking after your health. Swimming, especially, is known to be beneficial to asthma sufferers, as the warm, moist air above the water helps to loosen up the airways. However, as with most asthma advice, this is not entirely clear-cut, since chlorine in swimming pool water is known to trigger allergies in some people.

SCUBA DIVING

The idea of asthmatics attempting to scuba dive is sometimes greeted with horror, but it's by no means entirely out of the question. A 1994 survey showed that 4 per cent of people scuba diving as a hobby in Britain are asthmatic. **However if your asthma is triggered by the cold, by emotion or by exercise, you will not be allowed to scuba dive.** Dr Patrick Farrell is Vice-Chairman, UK Sport Diving Medical Committee, and he has helped to draw up the UK Standard for Asthmatic Divers. In Britain, asthmatics who follow these guidelines probably face no greater risk than normal divers. **However, scuba diving as a hobby is quite different from commercial and military diving, which exclude anyone with any asthma history.**

People whose asthma is likely to be triggered by aspects of scuba diving should not dive because:

- If you have an asthma attack underwater and you panic, you will use up your air supply too quickly and must surface.

- If you have an asthma attack underwater, you may not be able to surface unaided.

- In extreme cases, the high-pressure air that you are breathing can get trapped in the fine bronchioles of your airways, due to inflammation higher up the tubes. This can lead to pulmonary barotrauma (damage to the lungs because of air pressure) and air embolism (bubbles of air in the blood which can cause severe organ damage).

ASTHMA MEDICATION AND COMPETITIVE SPORT

Asthmatics whose sporting prowess takes them through to local, national or international competitions must seek advice from the sport's governing body on the medications they are allowed to take. For example, the International Olympic Committee Medical Commission has introduced mandatory reporting of all medication used for asthma to the appropriate medical officers or governing bodies. This is to ensure good treatment for asthmatics, and also to avoid the abuse of medication. The over-riding principle is that concerns about obeying the drug rules do not interfere with good asthma management.

Under International Olympic Committee rules, only two beta-agonists (relievers) are permitted: Bricanyl (terbutaline) and Ventolin (salbutamol). These are only to be taken using inhalers. Some athletes, under the misconception that this type of medication increases the availability of oxygen in the body, have been known to misuse relievers. In particular their use by non-asthmatics has become popular in many sports, and so there are some restrictions on use of reliever inhalers. For example, swimmers needing to use their relievers are required to leave the poolside, administer the treatment, and recover before returning to the pool to swim.

Inhaled corticosteroids such as Becotide, Flixotide and Pulmicort are all permitted for use by competitors in sporting competitions. In many sports asthmatics are required to register their treatments with the governing body medical officer. If, following a drugs test, salbutamol, terbutaline or corticosteroids are detected, the analytical report may be checked against the register of asthmatics. Similar reporting requirements have been introduced by many sports.

Further information on this is available from the Sports Council (see Useful Addresses).

To help prevent exercise-induced asthma, many asthmatics take a puff of their reliever inhaler just before a sports session. Cold air can trigger asthma, particularly during exercise when you are inhaling more frequently and more deeply than usual. This over-dries the surfaces of the airways and causes irritation. To overcome this problem, simply wear a scarf around your neck and over your mouth, or postpone your outdoor exercise until the air warms up a little.

If you experience asthma symptoms during sport, you will gain nothing by struggling on. There may be other trigger factors acting on your airways and the best course of action is to stop the sporting session, take a puff of reliever, and rest.

If you have had an acute asthma attack, particularly if you have had a course of oral steroids, you will need to withdraw from all sporting activity until you are fully recovered.

TRAVEL

Most people find travel stressful to some extent but an asthmatic has additional worries. You may well ask yourself: What if I have an attack in a foreign country? Will they know what to do?

Being prepared for such problems may help alleviate the stress – *they* may not know what to do about asthma, but *you* do. This means taking a good supply of reliever and preventative medication, a peak flow meter, and a spacer if you use one.

Some asthmatics who tend to have bad attacks will occasionally be prescribed prednisolone tablets, and may even have been advised by their doctors to carry an emergency supply. This supply *must* be taken with you when travelling. It is also important to pack your Asthma Management Plan (as described in Chapter 6) so that you can monitor your condition and adjust your medication accordingly. Carry all your medications, delivery devices and information as hand luggage.

You also need to consider your holiday environment. For example, if your asthma is triggered by the presence of animals, a pony trekking holiday *might* be a problem. On the other hand, you could anticipate the problems and take sensible precautions. Wearing a dust mask might enable you to groom the horses safely, especially if you use a reliever at the first sign of any wheeziness. Just before and during such a holiday you could increase your daily dosage of preventative medication to counteract the increased asthma triggers you are likely to encounter.

If you are in doubt about whether a particular holiday would be suitable for you, discuss with your doctor or asthma nurse the possibility of revising your Asthma Management Plan to take your holiday environment into account.

An asthmatic needs a holiday as much as the next person. Indeed many asthmatics report improvements in their asthma symptoms when they are on holiday. This could be due to the absence of stress, or the fact that you are breathing cleaner or warmer air. Certainly being an asthmatic should not, except in extreme or unusual cases, prevent you from going on holiday. On the contrary, a holiday may well help to calm your airways and so improve your asthma status.

Coping With Asthma At Work

Some jobs involve exposure to substances known to trigger or even induce asthma. Occupational asthma, as this is known, can be a serious problem. It is thought that about 200,000 people in the western world suffer from occupational asthma, and a further 500,000 may have asthma that is made worse by their work. Occupational asthma is therefore likely to be a major cause of work-related illness.

More than 200 substances have been reported as triggers for occupational asthma.

In the UK, the Department of Social Security publishes a list of substances which can cause asthma, and the jobs in which they are found. These are:

- **Isocyanates** – used for making plastics, foam, synthetic inks, paints and adhesives.

- **Platinum salts** – used in platinum refining workshops and some laboratories.

- **Acid anhydride and amine hardening agents, including expoxy resin curing agents** – used in a wide variety of industries, including adhesives, plastics, moulding resins and surface coatings.

- **Fumes produced by the use of rosin as a soldering flux** – mainly found in the electronics industry.

- **Proteolytic enzymes** – used in the manufacture of biological washing powders, as well as the baking, brewing, fish, silk and leather industries.

- **Animals including insects and other arthropods or their larval forms** – sometimes used for research, education, in laboratories, pest control and fruit cultivation.

- **Dust from barley, oats, rye, wheat or maize, or meal or flour made from such grain** – may be found in the baking or flour milling industries. Workers on farms may also be exposed to these dusts.

- **Antibiotics** – workers involved in their manufacture may be at risk.

- **Cimetidine** – used in the manufacture of cimetidine tablets (used in the treatment of gastric and duodenal ulcers).

- **Wood dust** – carpenters, joiners, papermill and sawmill workers may all be exposed to this.

- **Ispaghula powder** – used in the manufacture of bulk laxatives.

- **Castor bean dust** – merchant seamen, laboratory workers and felt makers may be exposed to this.

- **Ipecacuanha** – used in the manufacture of ipecacuanha tablets (a purgative and emetic).

- **Azodicarbonamide** – used as a blowing agent in the manufacture of expanded foam plastics used for wall-coverings, floor coverings, insulation and packaging materials.

- **Glutaraldehyde** – used for work in hospitals, laboratories, cooling towers and leather tanning.

- **Persulphate salts and henna** – hairdressers and those involved in the manufacture of hair products may be at risk.

- **Crustaceans** – workers exposed to crustaceans, fish or their products in the food processing industry may be at risk.

- **Reactive dyes** – mainly found in the dyeing, printing and textile industries.

- **Soya beans** – workers in the soya bean processing industry may be at risk.

- **Tea dust** – workers in the tea processing industry may be at risk.

- **Green coffee bean dust** – workers in the coffee processing industry may be at risk.

- **Fumes from stainless steel welding** – mainly found in metal working industries.

- **Any other sensitising agent** encountered at work.

This list refers only to British employment practices. The useful addresses section at the back of the book lists asthma organisations worldwide which will be able to give out relevant information about occupational asthma in other countries.

It may be possible to claim benefits if your asthma has been caused by exposure to certain substances in your workplace. In the UK, the procedure for doing this is outlined in a package obtainable from the Department of Social Security.

Avoiding exposure to these asthma-triggering substances can dramatically reduce occupational asthma, so it is in the interests of both employer and employee to take strict precautions when such substances are around. All workers should be protected against these substances, since there is evidence that anyone, not just people with an atopic tendency, can develop occupational asthma.

The good news is that companies are becoming more aware of the environment in which they place their workers. A good example of this is the trend towards non-smoking offices. The proven effects of passive smoking, and the likelihood of demands for compensation by those whose health has been endangered by it, are major factors in influencing employers to ban smoking in the workplace.

Having asthma may affect your choice of career, depending on the severity of your condition and how well it is managed. Some occupations exclude asthmatics, although perhaps not as many as you might think. The box below lists some of the most obvious occupations which would pose problems for an asthmatic. The information given refers to British companies and organisations. Recruitment practices may vary in other countries.

- **The Royal Air Force:** An asthmatic cannot join the RAF if he or she has had asthma symptoms or has taken asthma medication in the previous four years.

- **The Royal Navy:** An asthmatic cannot join the Royal Navy if he or she has had asthma medication in the previous four years.

- **The British Army:** An asthmatic cannot join the British Army if he or she has had asthma symptoms or has taken asthma medication in the previous four years.

- **The Police Force:** If you have had childhood asthma but have been clear of symptoms in adulthood you may be able to join the Police Force. Each individual is medically examined and judged on his or her own merits.

- **The Fire Brigade:** There are no specific guidelines concerning asthmatics, but it is essential that firefighters have a high level of aerobic fitness. Regulations specify that applicants should have no physical abnormality and should not be suffering from any disease.

- **The London Ambulance Service:** There is no blanket exclusion of asthmatics. Each case is assessed individually.

- **The Royal National Lifeboat Institution:** Some lifeboat crews do contain asthmatics. Each case is decided on its own merits by a doctor.

Having asthma certainly shouldn't prevent you from applying for most jobs, especially as many companies now have equal opportunities policies. If you can demonstrate that your asthma is well controlled and does not significantly affect your life, then being asthmatic should not lessen your chances of getting the job. British Airways, for example, considers each application on its merits and aims to allow the asthmatic to lead as normal a life as possible while avoiding exposure to environments which might provoke an attack.

As an asthma sufferer, you also have a responsibility to maintain your own good health. Instead of gamely struggling in to the office with a heavy cold, you should focus on recovering from the cold quickly, so that it does not *go onto your chest* and trigger an asthma attack. The body can fight the cold virus if you give it the resources to do so: rest is the most important of these. Influenza (flu) can also trigger an asthma attack. Doctors recommend that asthmatic patients have an annual flu vaccination, in order to lessen the chances of suffering from flu and then a prolonged attack of asthma. A vaccination should also lessen your chances of having to take time off work because of illness.

The responsibility to ensure that your asthma is properly managed lies with you, under the guidance of your doctor or asthma nurse. If this partnership is working successfully, then the answer to the question 'How will asthma affect my life?' can only be 'It won't – unless you let it . . .'

9

THE EMOTIONAL AND PSYCHOLOGICAL ASPECTS OF ASTHMA

Over the past 20 years, numerous studies have demonstrated that psychological factors play an important part in asthma management, and may even have an influence on whether or not people die from asthma. These factors include an unhappy home life, depression, panic, not co-operating with treatment, ignoring asthma symptoms, excessive emotion, and the effects of separation and bereavement.

It is reassuring to know that there are therapies and approaches that have proved beneficial in treating the psychological problems associated with asthma. This chapter identifies these psychological problems and discusses the treatments available to assist both carers and asthma sufferers in managing them effectively. **None of these psychological therapies are to be undertaken without your doctor's advice.**

Family Relationships

Children have to rely on their parents in many ways. They need to be cared for and nurtured and especially, need closeness and affection. If this closeness and affection is denied, they can become stressed, insecure and unstable. Asthma can be a frightening and lonely illness. It is important to know that those closest to you will be able to deal effectively with any potentially life-threatening situation, and that they can do so while remaining in control.

During the toddler stage, when a child first learns how to separate from his parents, the child's asthma may lead some parents to be over-protective. Other parents, in contrast, may not be able to cope with the child's neediness. As it is usually the mother who has the most contact with the child, her anxiety may sow the seeds of an anxiety disorder later on because of the child's increased sense of vulnerability.

A child needs a parent to be responsive to his need for dependence and at the same time responsive to his need to break away on his own. It is important for parents to identify these needs in their children and try to achieve a balance between dependence and independence.

It is entirely understandable that mothers, fathers and siblings sometimes react emotionally to a child's asthma. They too are frightened. It is not always easy to appear calm, patient and in control of the situation. Also, life must continue for the rest of the family. Brothers and sisters, especially, must be treated as equally as possible, since giving constant attention to the asthmatic child could lead to sibling rivalry and jealousy. The asthmatic child can be confused by the conflicting emotions expressed by his family, and will feel guilty as well as anxious about his illness.

Asthma can be a highly stressful disease both for parents and for asthma sufferers. Parents are more likely to develop a negative emotional attitude – either critical or over-protective – towards their child if the attacks occur frequently. This negative emotional attitude may create a stressful family environment which in itself can trigger the child's asthma. Asthmatic children in such an environment are less likely to co-operate in taking their medication. This pattern of negative parent-child interaction will make it more difficult for the parents to motivate their child to co-operate with the treatment. **Non-co-operation will increase the probability of recurring asthma attacks.**

Here are some typical examples of negative interaction in a stressed family environment:

- **Criticism** – 'You forgot to take your inhaler to school again. You expect me to remember everything for you.'

- **Negative solution** – 'I won't take you out until you calm down.'

- **Justification** – 'I didn't ask you to go out and play football when it was so cold; it's your fault you became so wheezy.'

- **Disagreement** – 'No I don't think you should have a hamster.'

Certain triggers may mean that asthmatic children are not allowed to do all the things they like doing. For example, they may have to avoid animal fur, despite liking pets very much; they may also have to stop in the middle of physical exercise, although they would like to continue. Parents need to find ways of presenting these limitations in a positive light, or the children may rebel and again fail to co-operate with their asthma medication.

Here are some examples of responding positively to common problems:

- 'We can leave a note on the fridge to help us to remember to put your inhaler in your school bag.'

- 'Just concentrate on your breathing. I'm here for you. We can go out as soon as you feel calmer.'

- 'We can always find some indoor sports for you to do when the weather is really cold.'

- 'It's not a good idea for you to have a hamster but you could have a guinea pig or a rabbit – they live outdoors.'

Family attitudes and responses to asthma can have a very positive influence on how an asthmatic child copes with their illness. A loving, supportive attitude, together with a well-informed understanding of treatment, can reduce the frequency and severity of the sufferer's asthma.

FAMILY THERAPY

Referral for family therapy is usually made through your doctor. In family therapy a professional therapist helps the family deal with their interactive problems. The therapy aims to make attitudes less rigid, improve the way in which families communicate, and deal with such issues as over-protectiveness. This sort of therapy has a positive effect on asthma, helping the family to:

- Manage both the circumstances that can trigger asthma and the various stresses produced by asthma itself.

- Behave calmly and make good use of medical services during severe asthma attacks.

- Improve their communication, so they have a better understanding of one another's needs.

Depression

A moderately depressed person lacks motivation, has less energy than usual, and may experience difficulty with concentration and memory. A severely depressed person may lack the motivation and energy to care for themselves, and may have difficulty interacting and functioning normally in their work and social situations. They may feel overwhelmingly helpless and hopeless.

An asthma sufferer may be depressed for many reasons, such as marital problems, work problems or any number of problems that cause people to become depressed. It is also possible that his asthma is making him depressed, particularly if it is poorly controlled and is interfering with his life. He may be wheezing during the night, not sleeping well and finding it difficult to cope during the day. He may have had one or two quite severe attacks during which he thought he would die. It is not unusual to be depressed after the trauma of such an episode.

If a person is suffering from asthma and depression at the same time, regardless of whether or not one caused the other, the two conditions seem to make each other worse. This means that the depression exacerbates the asthma, and, conversely, the asthma exacerbates the depression, so that the combined effect is greater than that of the two conditions acting separately.

The depressed asthmatic will probably fail to take his medication correctly, thus exposing himself to the risk of a severe asthma attack. He may also fail to react promptly to the early symptoms of an asthma attack, further compounding the risk.

Asthmatics with depression often find it difficult to express their emotions, and instead complain of physical ailments. The symptoms of 'masked' depression may include persistent complaints such as a chronic cough or breathing difficulties, rather than recognisable signs of depression. This means that the asthma sufferer is treated for the physical ailments but not for the depression which is the main problem.

If a depressed asthmatic adult has difficulty expressing their feelings to a doctor, it must be even harder for a child. The parent or carer must be perceptive and sensitive to signs of depression in a young child, such as being withdrawn and tearful, bedwetting and even refusing to go to school. Young children do not possess the maturity or vocabulary to express the desperation they are feeling. The parent must be patient and, above all, loving, caring and supportive.

TREATMENT OF DEPRESSION

For an asthmatic who is depressed, there are several strategies that can be adopted, and it is important for the asthma sufferer to work with his doctor to find the one most suited to his own needs.

Counselling may help the depressed asthmatic to solve the problems that are causing his depression. For example, counselling could enable him to find a way of resolving a conflict at work.

Another reason for his depression may be that his asthma is poorly controlled, and therefore restricting his life. In this case, adequate asthma medication may restore him to good health.

In other cases, anti-depressant medication can be very helpful when it is used appropriately. The doctor will know which anti-depressants are suitable for asthma sufferers.

Whichever treatment is chosen, it is important to monitor the asthmatic's response. Doctors can play a major role in educating asthmatics about the effects of medication, in monitoring the use of medication, and in providing support and counselling.

Anxiety And Panic Attacks

A *panic attack* is an episode of acute anxiety in which the heart beats rapidly and sweating occurs. The person may be confused and fear that he is about to die. It is usually accompanied by a breathing pattern called *hyperventilation* in which the breathing is deep and fast. *Panic disorder* is a condition that features recurrent, brief panic attacks, usually occurring about twice a week.

There are several factors in a person's background that may make them more likely to develop panic attacks or a panic disorder:

• Other members of the family having panic attacks or a panic disorder.

• Anxiety in other family members.

• A protracted and debilitating illness in a parent.

• Trauma during childhood, e.g. seeing someone dying or witnessing a serious accident in which a person is injured.

• Separation trauma, e.g. being hospitalised (which is quite likely for an asthmatic whose asthma is poorly controlled).

- Experiencing negative emotions, such as depression, as a result of poorly controlled asthma.

In some asthmatics, their asthma is the primary cause of their panic attacks. Asthmatics, quite naturally, have a heightened awareness of what is happening to their bodies, particularly when they feel an attack is imminent. Because of this they sometimes experience panic attacks when they mistakenly assume the symptoms they are experiencing will lead to a severe asthma attack. The frequency and severity of attacks among this group of asthma sufferers is strongly related to how well their asthma is controlled.

An asthma sufferer is more likely to panic when he is alone and focusing on his breathing, aware that there is no one at hand to reassure and calm him, and if necessary call for emergency assistance.

In other asthmatics, the panic attacks are caused, not by their asthma, but by other stress-inducing situations, such as being in a crowded shop, or being in an aeroplane. These are situations in which the person does not feel in control. The stress of the panic attack then triggers asthma, which in turn exacerbates the asthma sufferer's panic.

TREATMENT OF PANIC ATTACKS

During the panic attack itself, it is important to be calm and reassuring with the asthma sufferer, and to make sure the asthma is being correctly treated. An asthma attack and hyperventilation can appear quite similar. When a person hyperventilates they usually also complain of feeling breathless. Even doctors can have difficulty in distinguishing between hyperventilation and an asthma attack. **If you are in any doubt at all, seek help urgently.**

The treatment for panic attacks depends on the cause. If it is asthma that is triggering the panic, then the first step is to control the asthma properly with reliever medication. If the asthma sufferer is still having episodes of panic caused by the stress and fear of having asthma, then a psychological treatment called cognitive therapy may be appropriate.

COGNITIVE THERAPY

There are three stages in cognitive therapy. With the help of a doctor or a trained therapist, cognitive therapy helps asthma sufferers to:

- Identify how they view their condition.

- Recognise their fears.

- Look at ways of resolving their fears, so that they can anticipate and deal effectively with asthma or panic attacks in the future.

If the panic attacks are caused by stressful situations other than asthma, then behavioural therapy may be appropriate. It is also worth considering certain complementary therapies that promote relaxation and breathing control, such as the Alexander Technique and Yoga. (These and many other therapies are discussed in Chapter 10.)

BEHAVIOURAL THERAPY

Behavioural therapy also has three stages:

- The asthma sufferer is encouraged to put himself in

the situation that causes the panic, e.g. being in a crowded, stuffy atmosphere, riding on a train, or having to attend a social function.

- He is told that avoiding these situations will make his panic disorder worse and increase his subsequent fear of being exposed to potentially panic-inducing situations.

- He will be taught techniques to use during exposure to the feared situation. These will include breathing exercises (slow, deep breathing), and relaxation methods.

Asthmatics and their carers must first seek advice from their doctor before embarking on any psychological treatments.

Non-co-operation With Treatment

Non-co-operation (also known as poor compliance) is self-defeating, and can be very dangerous. Poor compliers often lack knowledge about asthma. Some asthmatics are not sufficiently aware of, or may ignore, the trigger factors that could exacerbate their asthma. Likewise, even well-informed asthmatics can be lax in their use of medication. However it is clear that poor compliance cannot be attributed to carelessness and lack of knowledge alone.

Poor compliers may face a significant deterioration in their quality of life because of asthma symptoms. They may have to withdraw from sporting and social activities, and may therefore feel inadequate. Children, in particular, express anger, fear and frustration at their condition because of the continual threat of sudden attacks, and the restrictions their asthma may place on their freedom to play. Understandably, asthma sufferers often feel some degree of bitterness and resentment.

They may express such sentiments as:

- 'Why me?'

- 'Asthma is ruining my life.'

- 'I am a prisoner of this disease.'

- 'I wish I could do the things everyone else takes for granted.'

- 'I feel like a misfit, the child that no one wanted in their team.'

For much of the time some asthma sufferers are largely free of symptoms and they may convince themselves that they are as fit and healthy as the next person. This category of asthmatic might choose to take prior medication on some public occasions, but not when they are alone. They often perceive their condition as being a social stigma, and fail to discuss their needs openly and honestly with carers and friends.

Some asthma sufferers may deny that they are ill. This behaviour pattern is known as *denial* (refusal to admit the reality or existence of something). If they take medication, they are admitting they are ill. So they refuse to take it. Denial may be due to problems the asthmatic has with pride and self-esteem which may be dented by having an 'illness'.

The long-term asthmatic may eventually come to comply with his treatment as a result of repeated asthma attacks. However this may not be true of young adults and children, for whom body image and social stigma are often of overriding concern.

Nowadays asthma sufferers and carers are expected to be

increasingly independent and responsible for their own health management. This is very difficult, given that the environment, with its many triggers, is variable and uncontrollable. Asthmatics might ask themselves about the symptoms they experience, and how these may vary and under what circumstances. What mood are they in today? What is the air quality like and what triggers are likely to affect their asthma today? Taking all these factors into account, should they attempt to cope on their own, with or without drugs, with or without support, or with the help of professionals? They must learn to be responsible for their illness and be able to assess when to ask someone for help.

Many sports personalities and athletes have succeeded in spite of their asthma, through regular and well-managed use of medication. Role models such as these should encourage asthmatics to comply with their medication.

Asthma involves significant risks which can be limited or even eliminated through regular medication and it is very important for the issue of non-compliance to be addressed. For doctors and asthma nurses, a good understanding of attitudes to asthma medication is crucial in encouraging good patient compliance. Likewise, it is the responsibility of asthma sufferers and their carers to be well informed about asthma and its treatment, so that the asthma sufferer can fulfil his potential and lead a safe and unrestricted life. **If you do not comply with your asthma medication, or the asthma sufferer you are responsible for does not, it is important for you to examine these issues urgently.**

Excessive Emotion

Many people experience strong emotions. These can be sad, such as during a bereavement, or happy, such as during the birth of a child. In asthmatics, these strong emotions can trigger an asthma attack.

Daniel would wake up nearly every night sweating profusely and, quite suddenly, be in the throes of an asthma attack. He would tell his mother that he had had the same nightmare again – the one where he was playing hide and seek and was locked in a cupboard which he could not open. He kept crying for help, but no one could hear or find him. It would take his mother some time to calm him down and reassure Daniel that she was always close and would come to him immediately.

Daniel's frequent nocturnal asthma attacks were apparently triggered by a recurring nightmare showing a fear of not being in control, followed by panic.

Stress can be a strong emotional trigger of asthma. And unresolved stress can lead to panic attacks or severe depression. As we have seen, both these conditions can trigger asthma in vulnerable people.

Many parents of asthmatic children have reported an increase in their child's wheezing when he has been crying, angry or excited. Wheezing is often reported as being provoked by laughter. At puberty many children appear to be 'growing out' of their asthma. However, for those children still experiencing asthma, particularly those with brittle asthma, the physical and emotional changes of puberty can cause immense stress which may trigger asthma. In addition, being acutely aware of body image, and wanting to establish their independence, they may not be taking their medication correctly.

TREATMENT OF EMOTION-TRIGGERED ASTHMA

If you know you are going to be exposed to a very stressful situation, or an episode of intense emotion, and your asthma has been triggered before under these circumstances, it is sensible to increase your preventative medication beforehand. Ideally, you will have discussed this type of situation with your doctor or asthma nurse when you drew up your Asthma Management Plan.

If you are faced with ongoing stress that you are finding difficult to handle, or you are depressed, or perhaps experiencing intense episodes of panic, discuss this with your doctor in order to identify the best psychological treatment or medication for you.

Asthma And School Attendance

Asthma may have a significant effect on school attendance and can also cause associated behavioural problems. A child whose asthma is well managed will cope with school life and control their asthma with relative ease. However, badly managed asthma may cause a child to miss a lot of schooling.

It is understandable for a parent to feel anxious when an asthmatic child gets ill. As a result, they will keep the child at home, either to overcome their asthma attack or to avoid making it worse. However, there is a tendency for the parents to become rather obsessive about potential asthma triggers and, in turn, project this attitude onto their child. This cycle of fear and protectiveness many create a negative downward spiral of poor school attendance and, consequently, poor performance. The child will see their academic performance as poor, and feel that they are lagging behind their peers. This can cause a 'fight or flight' response.

In the 'fight' mode, the asthmatic child will try to make up for the time lost through illness and ensure that their work is up to date. This usually means working additional hours at home, often with the support of a parent.

In the 'flight' mode, the asthmatic child will react against his perceived academic failure by engaging in a pattern of *refusal* behaviour and developing a disruptive attitude towards his peers and teachers. The child will refuse to do something, whether or not he is capable of achieving it, because he fears failing again, being teased by his classmates and told off by his teacher. In this way, a pattern of absenteeism, associated with fear of failure, low self-worth and lack of self-esteem, can be established. The parents of the asthmatic child may reinforce this behaviour by being overprotective and allowing the child to miss school. In such a situation, the child finds it progressively more difficult to break the vicious circle initially caused by his asthma.

This is a very sensitive issue for asthmatic children and their parents, and one that must be dealt with carefully, with support, and with an understanding of the child's depressed self-esteem. He should be given progressive goals that are achievable, thereby re-establishing his confidence. These steps should be monitored by both parent and teacher, and the child should be praised for all his efforts.

School life can be entirely normal for nearly all asthmatic children providing:

- The asthma sufferer is receiving the correct medication to control his asthma.

- There is good asthma awareness in the school.

- There is care and support for the asthma sufferer's particular needs.

- The asthma sufferer has good access to his medication.

Overcoming The Problems Through Self-management

Asthma self-management programmes are designed to teach asthmatics how best to manage their disease. These programmes have been shown to produce improved psychological adjustment to asthma, better co-operation in taking medication, greater competence in self-management of symptoms, and decreased use of medical services. Your doctor will provide the relevant information on how to get access to and benefit from the programmes. Such programmes tend to include:

- Providing information about asthma and asthma medications.

- Training and practice in trigger identification and avoidance.

- Training in self-assessment of asthma symptoms and in the use of peak flow meters to assess exacerbations in asthma and as a guide to taking medication or seeking medical care.

- Training in breathing techniques, posture, relaxation, and stress reduction.

- Using group and family therapy to reduce the fear and anxiety that often accompany the disease.

- Encouraging general healthy habits and attitudes.

For asthmatics to cope well with their asthma, they must have a good understanding of an often complex daily medication regime. They must also be able to distinguish between acute and maintenance medication, to increase or reduce doses appropriately, and to seek help when necessary.

Good self-management creates a feeling of well-being and removes hindrances and restrictions for asthma sufferers in everyday life.

10

COMPLEMENTARY THERAPIES

Nowadays schools teach about caring for the environment, and our children question the ethics of formerly accepted activities, such as eating meat or using fossil fuels. Popular books, such as *The Animals of Farthing Wood*, reflect these concerns:

> *In another field they saw more lifeless creatures: poisoned fieldmice and beetles, and pretty butterflies which had unavoidably been tainted with the death-dealing spray. Even bees, useful to humans, had ignorantly strayed into this area where only machines and the mathematical minds of men were permitted to hold sway. These innocent makers of honey had perished too ... 'I wonder,' mused Fox, 'Can humans always be right? It must need only a small error for them to put themselves at danger, using such terrifying materials.'*
>
> from *The Animals of Farthing Wood* by Colin Dann

In matters of health, assumptions are also being questioned and, as we become more widely informed, many people are starting to feel that conventional treatment is no longer the only answer. Conventional, or *allopathic* treatment, is based on the principle of treating a disease with opposition. For example, if there is an inflammation, it is treated with an anti-inflammatory medicine.

The word **holism** encapsulates the spirit of complementary therapies. Holism is the consideration of the complete person, both physically and psychologically. This means building up a detailed picture of the patient's needs and feelings before embarking on a course of treatment. It may well mean using a combination of complementary therapies. Holism promotes healing and well-being and encourages the patient to take part in his own healing through changes of attitude and lifestyle. So, in the spirit of the age, people are looking for alternatives, for less invasive ways of improving their health.

People may visit a complementary therapist for various reasons. They could be merely curious, following up the recommendations of friends, books or newspaper articles. Or they could be lacking in faith – in their own doctor, in his choice of treatment, or in conventional medicine generally. With asthma this lack of faith represents a serious problem. To avoid the risk of a full-blown attack, all but the mildest asthma *must* be treated with conventional medicine on a daily basis. If you think your doctor is not managing your asthma well, find another doctor who is asthma-aware.

However, many asthma sufferers ascribe their improved health to complementary therapies, and some of them can certainly be helpful. Stress and anxiety are known to be asthma triggers, and any *safe* treatment that alleviates these is worth considering. But the emphasis must definitely be on the word **safe**.

This chapter describes a number of complementary therapies, showing how they may be helpful and highlighting pitfalls to avoid. Always discuss with your doctor or asthma nurse any complementary therapies you are planning to use. Together, you will be able to assess the potential benefits or problems, and fit these therapies into your Asthma Management Plan.

You must make sure that your therapist is professionally qualified before starting treatment. Most complementary therapies have a professional society who will supply lists of their members, sometimes asking for a small fee to cover postage.

All complementary therapies should be used *alongside* the medication prescribed by your doctor, *not instead of it*. If your complementary therapist tells you to stop taking the medication your doctor has prescribed for your asthma, walk away.

Calming Therapies

The stresses and anxieties of life are known asthma triggers. Also, before and during an asthma attack, panic can set in. The asthmatic feels as if he is being starved of air (as if he were drowning). This makes him panic and, if uncontrolled, this panic can worsen the attack.

Safe therapies which help asthmatics to be calm and to relax are beneficial. In fact, of the published scientific studies on asthma and complementary therapies, those concerned with relaxation techniques have shown the best evidence of improving the health of asthmatics. Hypnosis and yoga seem to be particularly effective.

HYPNOSIS

A hypnotic state is one in which you are neither asleep nor awake but in a trance, brought about by a hypnotist. Most people can be put into a hypnotic state fairly easily. The hypnotist will then suggest ideas and give instructions to the patient, who will continue to concentrate on these ideas once he has been brought out of the hypnotic state.

In asthma, hypnotism may also involve looking at the issues behind the illness, such as emotional problems, and trying to disentangle the asthma symptoms from the causes of the asthma.

YOGA

Yoga was first practised in India as early as 3000 BC. It is a philosophical system, concerned with attaining union with the Universal Spirit. This is achieved by learning to control the mind, thus overcoming fear, pain and suffering. The practice of yoga includes learning *poses* (static or moving positions), breathing exercises, diet and meditation.

In the West, yoga classes tend to focus mainly on yoga as a form of exercise aiming to reduce stress. The combined effects of yoga poses, breathing exercises, relaxation and meditation help change our emotional state in order to release the stress in our bodies.

Breathing techniques are taught in yoga classes, and these are especially helpful for asthmatics. Yoga focuses on *diaphragmatic breathing* – breathing from low down in the back and stomach rather than from the upper chest. (This is also the type of breathing that singers learn.) Diaphragmatic breathing expands the lungs and enables you to absorb more oxygen.

MEDITATION

This is another ancient technique which can help relaxation. It is taught as an aspect of yoga, but may be practised separately. Meditation involves calming and quietening the mind, and thus brings about a calm state in the body.

RELAXATION

There are many techniques for relaxation, working separately or together on the mind and the body. The object of any relaxation method is to counterbalance the stresses and strains of everyday life, and enable us to stop, focus on ourselves and our tensions, and learn to release those tensions.

Generally, relaxation techniques are taught in quiet surroundings, where small groups of people learn to focus their minds on an image, a word, a sound or a single thought. You will be taught to *let go*, allowing tension and strain to escape. This may involve clenching and relaxing your muscles, slowly, from your toes to the top of your head. You will feel comfortable and secure, and after the relaxation you are likely to experience a sense of well-being and calm.

For asthmatics, a good relaxation technique is well worth acquiring. You may need to look at different relaxation methods in order to find one that suits you. Once learnt, such techniques can be used at any time and would be particularly helpful in controlling the panic and stress associated with an asthma attack.

Other Complementary Therapies

There are several other complementary therapies which some asthma sufferers find helpful.

ACUPUNCTURE

Acupuncture has an impressive pedigree. It is part of an ancient system of medicine which began in China over 2,000 years ago.

Traditional acupuncture is based on the principle that our health depends on the body's life force flowing through it in a harmonious and balanced way. This force is called the Ch'i, and it contains the dual energy flows, Yin and Yang. These two are opposites and are found within the human body and everywhere in the universe, complementing each other.

The aim of acupuncture is to restore harmony between these equal and opposite qualities of Ch'i and, in doing so, to enable the body to fulfil its innate self-healing ability. Within the body are meridians (channels beneath the skin) along which the body's energy flows. Acupuncture is concerned with regulating this flow of energy and so restoring harmony to the body.

Tests have proved that the brain releases *endorphins* (pain-relieving morphine-like substances) when acupuncture points on the body are stimulated. This may explain why acupuncture has been used instead of anaesthesia in some surgical operations.

An acupuncturist tries to discover the area of disharmony within the body by observing and talking to the patient. He will usually inspect the patient's tongue, and feel for several pulses on each wrist. Then he will decide where to apply the acupuncture needles.

Fine needles are used to pierce the skin at specific points above the meridians. This is a fairly painless technique. The practitioner may combine the insertion of the needles with *moxibustion* (burning a small cone of dried herbs on or near the skin). This feels pleasantly warm.

Acupuncture claims to be beneficial when an organ's function is impaired (as opposed to cases where the organ is diseased or damaged). As asthma is due to impaired function of the airways in the lung, acupuncture is said to be helpful for asthmatics.

THE ALEXANDER TECHNIQUE

The Australian F. Matthias Alexander founded this technique. The publication of his book, *The Use of Self*, in 1932 led to worldwide interest in his system for improving people's lives.

Alexander, an actor, evolved his technique in order to improve his vocal delivery. He observed that when he began to deliver a line his posture altered and his voice weakened. So he worked on observing his posture and making changes. With them, his vocal delivery improved. Eventually

Alexander developed his method for retraining the body, particularly in the carriage of the neck and head.

The Alexander Technique is now taught through a series of lessons in which the teacher guides the pupil to focus on his customary posture, movement and balance. He then learns how to change his posture and the way in which he uses his body. Through these changes, tension is released, the body is realigned and natural balance is improved. Pupils must then practise regularly to acquire the discipline of using the technique for themselves.

The Alexander Technique claims to be effective in alleviating chronic conditions, including breathing disorders and asthma. It is usually taught on day courses.

REFLEXOLOGY

Reflexology is another method of treatment which can trace its origins back to the ancient Chinese. In the 1930s it was most famously described by an American, Eunice Ingham, who based her theories on a work called *Zone Therapy*. Reflexology is now taught and practised widely, and is considered to be both an art and a science.

Reflexology is based on the theory that energy zones run through the body, and that the body can be mapped out on the feet, with each foot corresponding to one side of the body. The inside curve of the foot matches the curve of the spine, and all parts of the body are represented within this 'foot map'. Because the whole body is depicted here, the reflexologist is able to treat the patient holistically.

Reflexologists believe that ten energy zones run through the body from head to toe, embracing all organs and parts of the body. By stimulating a zone marker in the foot, they claim to influence that entire zone throughout the body.

A reflexology session begins with detailed discussion of the patient's medical history, followed by an examination of the feet, and then the massage. This is usually given with the side and end of the thumb, and all areas on both feet will be massaged. The areas that correspond with the parts of the body that are giving problems will sometimes be tender during the treatment. The specific reflexology area for treating asthma is the ball of the foot.

After a session of reflexology the patient may undergo a *healing crisis*, due to the release of impurities into his system. This reaction may include headaches and nausea, and can last about 24 hours. The reflexologist would see the experience of a healing crisis as a good thing, since it would indicate that the treatment was having an effect.

HOMOEOPATHY

Homoeopathy is a system of healing which has been established for around 200 years. In 1796 Samuel Hahnemann, a German doctor, discovered a different approach to curing the sick which he called homoeopathy, after the Greek words meaning 'similar suffering'.

Hahnemann's theories were based on the ancient idea that there are two ways of dealing with ill-health – the way of opposites and the way of similars. Allopathic medicine uses opposites; homoeopathy uses similars.

Homoeopathy aims to assist the body's natural tendency to heal itself. It recognises that all symptoms of ill-health represent disharmony in the body. It is this disharmony that needs to be addressed, so that the body's own healing powers are stimulated to deal with the symptoms. Homoeopathic treatment is often referred to as treating *like with like*, giving a medicine which matches the patient's symptoms in a minute and highly diluted dose.

Students of classical homoeopathy – based on the teachings and philosophy of Hahnemann – undertake three or four years of study in which aspects of health and disease are covered from both a medical and a homoeopathic point of view. Nowadays it is not uncommon for doctors in conventional medicine to work in association with homoeopathic doctors, sometimes even as a part of the same medical practice. Also, just as in conventional medicine some health centres offer specialist asthma clinics, so some homoeopaths also offer asthma clinics.

A visit to a homoeopathic asthma clinic is likely to involve the following. You begin with a short consultation before deciding whether to opt for the treatment. For an adult a full appointment lasts about one and a half hours. There will probably be an extensive questionnaire about your asthma to fill in. This will try and find out such information as what makes your breathing better or worse, what you do during an asthma attack, how you feel about your asthma and so on. You will be asked about your family's medical history, your relationships, stresses and attitudes to life. The object of this investigation is to find a homoeopathic remedy that takes account of your whole symptom picture.

Homoeopathic remedies are made from plant substances, from minerals, are of animal origin, or are from disease substances. These substances are highly diluted, and are usually taken in tablet form. You will be asked to take these tablets as prescribed, and then return to the clinic after two weeks. During that time you are usually able to telephone and receive further advice if necessary.

Asthmatics could expect to be taking homoeopathic remedies for up to six months: improvement may not happen immediately. If real improvement has taken place it is not usually necessary to continue taking homoeopathic remedies, but you can resume the tablets at a later date if the symptoms return.

If you are taking homoeopathic medicine you should not abandon your inhalers, even if you are feeling an improvement. It could be dangerous to do this.

After homoeopathic treatment you may experience one of several changes. You may feel well and hopeful, or your symptoms may worsen for a while. This would be seen as a sign that the treatment was having an effect. You may develop a cold, a rash or another form of discharge which would indicate that the system was cleansing itself. Old symptoms may reappear. The homoeopath would need to know about any of these.

Homoeopathy does seem to help some asthmatics, particularly children and adults who have not had the disease for very long. Homoeopathy can be effective quickly, but it can also take time. It can work alongside conventional medicine, and the professional body certainly recommends that you maintain contact with your doctor, and that you inform him if you are being treated homoeopathically.

Like other complementary therapies, there are few official restrictions on who can claim to be a homoeopath. If you are considering homoeopathy as an asthma treatment, it is important that you see a registered homoeopath. These homoeopaths practice in accordance with a Code of Ethics and Practice, have professional insurance, and have passed stringent academic and clinical assessments before being admitted to the register (see Useful Addresses).

HERBAL MEDICINE

Herbal medicine is the use of plant remedies to treat disease. Man has been treating himself in this way for centuries, and herbalism remains the most widely practised form of medicine in the world.

Herbalists believe that the balance of the plant's healing content is contained in whole components of the plant, such as the leaves or the roots, or indeed the whole plant. They feel that isolating one chemical from the plant and using it to treat disease may be counter-productive, as a plant can contain hundreds of other chemicals which assist the healing process or indeed allow it to happen.

Conventional medicine takes a different approach. Sometimes a single chemical may be isolated from a plant, purified, and then used as a medicine. Alternatively, a medicine may be totally synthetic, its composition being precisely tailored for a particular function.

An example of this contrast between the two disciplines is in the use of ephedrine. This is a natural bronchodilator which comes from the herb *Ephedra sinica* and is used in herbal medicine to treat asthma. Ephedrine has many side-effects, including the raising of blood pressure. Salbutamol is a synthesised alternative to ephedrine, designed to be inhaled and to cause bronchodilation with minimal side-effects. However, herbalists would maintain that if ephedrine is administered as a component of the pure extract of the ephedra plant, the side-effects will be negated by other elements of the plant extract.

Using herbal remedies alongside conventional medication can have a fatal outcome. For example, digitalis comes from the foxglove plant and is highly effective in the treatment of heart disease. The purified form of digitalis used in conventional medicine is called digoxin. However, as any fan of Agatha Christie's detective novels will know, if digitalis is taken in uncontrolled doses it is a deadly poison. If a patient decided to seek treatment from his herbalist as well as his doctor and was given both foxglove and digoxin, the outcome could be fatal.

Mixing herbal remedies with conventional medicines can be extremely dangerous. *Always* tell your doctor if you are taking any herbal remedies. And if you are already taking a conventional medicine, do not start taking a herbal remedy without first consulting your doctor.

It would be wonderful to get better without taking endless drugs, and using a method that retains an element of mystery in an age where science tries to explain everything. Some complementary therapies cannot be scientifically supported, but many people will testify that they are of benefit.

Only seek the advice of a professional complementary therapist. In addition, always discuss any complementary therapies you are using with your doctor, and follow his advice about your asthma medication.

11

PARENTS AND ASTHMA

'It's all my fault. I get hayfever and I've passed it on to her and now she is going to have asthma for the rest of her life . . .'

This is a common response from parents whose children have been diagnosed as asthmatic. You may feel guilty, especially if a pattern of asthma and allergies runs through your family and you feel responsible for passing it on. If you suspect asthma in your child, these feelings of guilt may prevent you telling your doctor, for fear that your child will be labelled asthmatic. You may even subconsciously wish to deny that you suspect asthma, and therefore avoid the confirmation a doctor could give you.

You might also be frightened of the condition. It *is* frightening to see anyone struggling for breath – particularly when that person is your own child. But feeling this way is far more terrifying for your child, who assumes that breathing is automatic. To suddenly find yourself unable to breathe properly is a shock. It is therefore essential to reassure your child and show him that his parents are in control and can do something about the situation. This can be very difficult; you have to behave calmly, even though you may be feeling desperately worried. But realising how important it is for your child seems to give most parents the strength to stay in control.

So, as a parent, you have a central role in the management of your child's asthma – from the initial suspicion and first visit to the doctor, to daily monitoring and treatment. This management role may last for many years but if you can fulfil it effectively your asthmatic child will be able to live a normal life and achieve his full potential.

The most important tasks for a parent are:

- Taking your child to the doctor to be diagnosed.

- Being informed about asthma.

- Being able to cope if your child has an acute attack.

- Checking your child's inhalers.

- Eliminating triggers in your home.

- Checking your child's diet.

Taking Your Child To The Doctor

There are several warning signals which can be quite subtle and non-specific, but which may lead parents to wonder whether their children have asthma. These include a persistent irritating cough, particularly at night or first thing in the morning; what is commonly described as 'chestiness'; a reluctance to run around and join in games or sports; frequent courses of antibiotics; and, of course, wheezing. **If, when your child breathes out, there is at times a sound like a feeble bagpipe, he is likely to be asthmatic.** A good maxim for any concerned parent suspecting asthma is **if in doubt, refer to your doctor** – that's what he's there for.

If you suspect asthma, it is your job as a parent to describe precisely the symptoms to your doctor. Unfortunately, a few doctors are still not fully asthma-aware and this, coupled with parental unwillingness to accept the possibility of asthma, could colour the doctor's diagnosis. So, for a parent, it is essential to overcome anxiety and guilt about your child's asthma. Otherwise those feelings may influence the quality of treatment your child receives.

In the unlikely event of your doctor being unwilling to diagnose asthma, even though you are fairly sure that your child is asthmatic, you have every right to seek another opinion. Be persistent, and express any doubts you may have. After all, it is your child's welfare that is at stake. **More often than not, parental instinct, coupled with your love for your child, will lead to the most perceptive judgement of the problem.**

Try to identify those doctors who are particularly asthma-aware. Here you can tap into the local bush telegraph: parents of other asthmatic children will soon tell you which doctors to visit and which to avoid. **As a general rule, if a practice has an active asthma clinic, the doctors within that practice will be asthma-aware.**

Being Informed About Asthma

Parents need to be well informed about asthma. This is not a difficult task, and it is essential. You need to be confident in dealing with your child's medication, but also know when to call for help. Your child needs to sense that confidence, and be able to relax in the knowledge that you can deal with his condition effectively. A parent whose child is having an asthma attack **must stay calm**.

The most important part of good asthma management is continuous use of medication in the dosage specified by your doctor. The main medication is likely to be inhaled steroids (such as Becotide or Pulmicort) and your child may be advised to take them indefinitely.

Inhaled steroids are the most effective anti-inflammatory

agents we have, and they are the means by which asthma sufferers are prevented from having asthma attacks. Unfortunately, the word *steroid* can strike fear into the hearts of parents. However, it is important to remember that the normal dosage is **minimal**, because steroids are inhaled directly into the lungs and go to work immediately on the inflamed areas. Very little is absorbed into the bloodstream, and so other organs are unaffected. Parents may be concerned because they have heard of a link between steroids and growth suppression in children. However, inhaled steroids have been used for about 20 years, and there is no convincing evidence that, at normal dosages, they impair a child's growth. It is important to bear in mind that prevention is far better than emergency treatment. Your child's asthma should be suitably controlled at all times in order to minimise the possibility of an acute attack.

Properly managed, and with appropriate medication, almost all asthmatic children can be well and lead normal lives. But there is a very small group whose condition is difficult to control, and who do need exceptionally high dosages of inhaled steroids, such as two puffs of Becloforte four times a day.

These children will be under hospital-based specialist management. They *may* be subject to some growth suppression, due to the high dosages of inhaled steroids. Even so, most parents would probably feel that exchanging a centimetre or two in height was a reasonable price to pay for gaining control over a chronic and potentially life-threatening condition.

There is also a very small percentage (about 1–2 per cent) of asthmatic children whose condition still deteriorates at times, despite their medication. These children can be extremely difficult to manage, and asthma may interfere with their lifestyles. It is important that they are under the care of a hospital specialist, preferably one with a particular interest in asthma.

Coping With An Acute Attack

An acute attack is a very serious situation which requires immediate medical attention (see Chapter 7). The symptoms include:

- loud wheezing that lessens as the attack becomes more severe;

- recession (in-drawing of flesh between the ribs);

- inability to say more than a few words due to lack of breath;

- blue lips;

- intense withdrawal and concentration.

These symptoms are extremely distressing to both child and parent.

A parent, or anyone caring for a child displaying any of these symptoms, *must* call a doctor or an ambulance immediately. Your role in an acute asthma attack is to **keep calm**, reassure your child, keep **him calm** and treat him with reliever medication, such as Ventolin (salbutamol), repeatedly if necessary, until help arrives. Children have an acute sense of impending danger and this can easily be picked up from what people around them are saying. There are words and phrases of reassurance, and there are words and phrases of panic. Make sure you only use the reassuring ones when your child can hear you.

However it *is* essential to express panic on the phone in order to get proper treatment quickly. The key words are 'SEVERE ASTHMA ATTACK'. Make sure your child does not overhear you talking on the phone, as this knowledge could make him panic, and thus worsen the attack.

REASSURANCE	PANIC
Relax, you'll be fine.	He can't breathe.
Lots of children have asthma.	He's struggling for breath.
Don't worry, I know what to do.	The inhaler isn't working, what shall I do? Should I call the doctor? People
The doctor/hospital can make it better straight away.	die of asthma!
Don't worry, I'm here to help you.	

Checking Your Child's Inhalers

Here your role is supervisory: maintaining the inhalers and enabling your child to use them with confidence. The first point is to regularly check the use-by date. Inhalers can get past their best, in which case they need to be replaced promptly.

You should also check that the inhalers are working properly and that they are not clogged up. Inhalers should always have their caps on when not in use. An open inhaler lying around in the bottom of an over-stuffed school bag could easily be primed with a potentially dangerous object like a nut, crumbs, pieces of rolled-up paper, rubber, pencil shavings and so on. A child unwittingly taking these into his lungs through his inhaler could choke.

As we have already seen, asthma sufferers using MDIs, in which the medication is concealed within a metal canister, cannot tell how much medication remains. Although you can shake the canister and listen to the contents, this is not reliable. If you suddenly run out of your regular adrenaline-like reliever medication, your asthma can actually be exacerbated.

To overcome this problem, you should always ensure that you have a spare new inhaler, and request the repeat prescription as soon as your child starts the spare inhaler. In that way you will never experience the nightmare scenario of a badly asthmatic child puffing away at an empty inhaler and panicking when he receives no relief. There is a further, psychological aspect to this. The knowledge that he *can* use his inhaler the moment he feels his asthma coming on may diminish the actual need. **The golden rule is: always have spare inhalers.**

Away from home, an asthmatic child ought to be responsible for his own inhaler. Parents must ensure that he is well instructed in the correct use of his inhaler, and can identify the appropriate times to take it. **As long as he is able to use an inhaler properly, without supervision, it is essential that he keeps it with him at all times.**

It is highly likely that, away from home, nobody will observe the early stages of a child experiencing asthma. There is no blood, no rash, no high temperature. So your child needs his inhaler close at hand. If this means having one inhaler at the bedside, one in his schoolbag, another in his gym bag and another in his pocket, so be it. They are usually prescribed in pairs anyway. It would also be useful for the school to keep a reliever inhaler in the first aid box.

Before our school trip to the Lake District we knew that there were several asthmatics in the party. We were confident because of our asthma training, and the girls were well aware that they must always have their inhalers with them. But on the one occasion when a girl did have an attack we were out on a field trip.

And where was her inhaler? In her bag, back at the hotel. It was a sticky situation, but we all remained calm and got her back to the hotel as quickly as possible. We were shaken, though, because it could have been far more serious.

This child should not have been relying on the teachers to mollycoddle her. It was her condition and she should have been responsible for carrying her inhaler. In an ideal world, teachers will have been trained in asthma treatment and will understand how important it is to have inhalers on hand *at all times*. But in schools where there is less asthma-awareness, parents need to ensure that their children's inhalers are where they need them to be.

Many schools are equipped with spacers (see p. 47), to help with effective inhaler use. Both parents and children need to know how to use a spacer, and they should learn how to use it during *normal* breathing, not when the child is having an attack. As a parent, you could expand the familiarisation into a school asthma-awareness campaign, so that teachers and other pupils can be confident about asthma. To begin with, the class could be shown a spacer and an inhaler in action. In this way, parents can help to ease asthma-awareness into schools.

Eliminating Triggers

As already discussed, a vast range of triggers can cause the airways to become inflamed, thus exacerbating asthma. Parents can make the home a safer place for an asthmatic child by eliminating as many triggers as possible. The most common triggers of asthma in the home include house dust mites, animal skin (dander), pollen and moulds.

HOUSE DUST MITES

As we have seen, house dust mites are potent triggers of asthma in the home. They tend to congregate in bedrooms, which is where asthmatics often experience their worst symptoms. Parents must make a big effort to control their population.

Regular vacuuming will reduce the quantities of mites. There are vacuum cleaners on the market which claim to filter out all house dust mites, and using one of these may be reassuring. However, as most new vacuum cleaners feature high filtration, the accent should be on using an efficient machine rather than an expensive one. Look at your vacuum cleaner dispassionately: if there is a cloud of dust escaping from the back, it is unlikely to be filtering well.

Damp dusting, a practice widely used in hospitals, is another simple way of removing house dust mites. (Dusting with a dry cloth merely tends to send these tiny creatures up into the air.)

So the emphasis is on simple, commonsense measures:

- Vacuum regularly and effectively (including mattresses).

- Damp-dust thoroughly.

- Get rid of feather pillows and mattresses (or use allergen-proof covers).

- Keep wardrobe doors closed (so dust does not settle on clothes).

- Cut down on the number of soft toys in the bedroom. These harbour dust.

- Allow a regular flow of fresh air through the room (but not a blast of winter gale!).

ANIMAL DANDER

Just as humans shed their skin and leave a feast for the house dust mite, so do pets. Flakes of animal skin and tissue, known as dander, are deposited wherever a domestic animal goes. There is no advantage to the asthmatic in having a short-haired rather than a long-haired pet.

Here there is potential for a massive conflict between commonsense and emotion. In theory, asthmatics and animals should not live in the same house. In practice, the emotional effect of suddenly banishing a beloved friend could do more harm than good. So the simple commonsense rules are:

- Do not get any new pets.

- Never allow pets in bedrooms.

- Always groom pets out of doors.

- Try sending your pets to a friend or relative for two or three months. During that time the amount of animal dander in your home would reduce significantly. If your child's asthma is considerably better, you might have to make the decision not to allow the animals to return.

- Vacuum and dust thoroughly and regularly.

SMOKING

Cigarette smoke makes existing asthma much, much worse. It is a potent trigger. Furthermore, a child living in a house where people smoke is twice as likely to develop asthma. There are no half measures here. For the sake of your child's health, you *cannot* smoke in the house. Allow your children to breathe clean air in their own home and make every effort to prevent children from ever taking up smoking.

So you should aim to make your house as friendly as possible for the asthma sufferer but it should not become an obsession. You certainly need not feel shamed into buying every new product for which you are targeted by advertisers. Some may work for your child; some may not. Commonsense and simple precautions cost little – try them first.

Checking Your Child's Diet

If you are worried about your child's diet, you will be heartened to know that the trigger for his asthma is unlikely to be food or drink.

Occasionally cow's milk, eggs and nuts may be suspected, as well as food additives such as tartrazine and monosodium glutamate, but no specific trigger linking these foods has been isolated.

If you suspect that a particular food – say peanuts – is triggering asthma in your child, the obvious response is to eliminate that food from his diet. It is also essential to inform your child's school, in writing, of this problem.

If food or drink triggers are suspected but you are unsure which specific item is to blame, your child can be put onto an exclusion diet (see p. 68). You should not attempt this alone but should consult your doctor or asthma nurse. Exclusion diets are time-consuming and not wholly reliable, so you might justifiably feel that you would be better off looking elsewhere for the causes of your child's asthma.

Will Asthma Impair My Child?

Knowing that your child has asthma, and may have it for the rest of his life, is a frightening prospect for many parents. You need to believe that asthma will not be allowed to rule his life.

Properly managed, with well-informed parental involvement, most asthmatic children do lead normal lives.

However, a child who lacks confidence, because of ineffective medication and consequent ill-health, may seem impaired. He may be reluctant to take part in physical activities; he may be withdrawn; he may not want to go out to play. In short, his asthma may lead him to avoid things. This avoidance behaviour could lead to frequent absence from school, and poor educational performance.

A five-year-old girl's elbow was dislocated after she had been swung round by an adult. In abject misery the family looked on as the casualty nurse strapped her arm up. Thus treated, the little girl coped with her condition. The injured arm hurt, so she did not use it. It was as if the arm was no longer part of her. For two miserable days, the little girl ignored her arm and managed without it. When she returned to hospital, the pain had subsided and she was able to relax while the elbow was manipulated back into place. Within seconds, she took possession of her arm again, and was waving it about as if nothing had ever been wrong.

An asthmatic child copes in the same way. If he feels threatened by his condition, he will withdraw to a safer position. Once his condition is under control, he will confidently step out and revert to what he would normally be doing.

Without forcing your child to participate in any activity, you need to show him that he *can* elbow the asthma aside and get on with what he wants to do. With regular preventative medication, and with a reliever inhaler always at hand, an asthmatic child can keep active and healthy and participate fully in all aspects of life.

It might be helpful to compare asthma with short-sightedness, another common, everyday childhood condition:

- People who are short-sighted are not going to be 'cured': people with asthma are not (at least for the foreseeable future) going to be 'cured'.

- Glasses can correct the problem of short sight: inhalers can correct the problem of asthma.

- Short-sighted children may occasionally be teased but well-designed modern glasses can be the envy of friends: treatment for today's asthmatic children is far more effective than it used to be, and generally the population is more aware of the condition.

- Short-sighted children lead normal lives: asthmatic children lead normal lives.

So why has your child got asthma? And is it your fault? The answer is that he has asthma because something triggers it. He may have been genetically predisposed to asthma, but without the triggers the asthma would not occur. Since you can hardly shoulder the blame for all the pollution in the air we breathe, for all the animals in the world, for every dust mite, every piece of pollen or every cold virus, you can consider yourself 'not guilty'.

Having eliminated the guilt, you are free to consider the positive action you can take. As a parent you are best placed to ensure that your child's asthma is managed effectively. Who makes the difference between an asthmatic child leading a normal, full life, and an asthmatic child whose condition dominates and inhibits his life? His parents.

12

ASTHMA IN SCHOOLS

The fat boy stood by him, breathing hard.
'My auntie told me not to run,' he explained, 'on account
of my asthma.'
'Ass-mar?'
'That's right. Can't catch me breath. I was the only boy in
our school what had asthma . . .'
                    from *Lord of the Flies* by William Golding

If you were once an asthmatic child, and are reading this
because your son or daughter has just been diagnosed asthmatic, the good news is that general awareness of asthma has
progressed enormously since William Golding created the
character of Piggy, and the stigma attached to the disease is
fast fading. This is not surprising when you consider that
today nearly all schoolchildren have close experience of
asthma: a family member or friend may have asthma; they
may have heard of a well-known sports star with asthma; or
they may have asthma themselves.

For a child, asthma can be annoying, embarrassing,
painful and terrifying – all or any of these feelings are common. During an acute asthma attack, the asthma sufferer
may feel that he is going to die. At school it is particularly
important that someone knows that the child is suffering and
knows what to do about it, in order to make the child feel
confident that he will receive support.

Do Teachers Need To Know About Asthma?

At school the welfare of the child is in the hands of the teacher who is acting *in loco parentis* – in the place of the parents. To fulfil this responsibility, the teacher needs to be informed about anything that may influence the child's welfare.

If a child falls at school and breaks his leg, his teachers will treat him confidently, knowing not to move him, knowing that they have to keep him warm and comfortable, knowing that they have to call an ambulance. The teachers are informed about broken legs, enabling them to accurately assess the situation and take appropriate action.

As many as 20 per cent of schoolchildren are asthmatic, and up to half these children are undiagnosed; children who are persistently 'chesty' but whose parents or doctors have not yet connected the symptoms with asthma. Any day, any of these children could experience a serious asthma attack. There is every chance that this will happen at school and, if so, the teacher can only take appropriate action if he is informed about asthma.

What Should A Teacher Do When A Pupil Has An Asthma Attack?

During a vigorous football practice on a cold afternoon, young James slows down, drops to the ground and seems to be gasping for air. What do you do? If you have no basic asthma training, the first thing you will probably do is panic. James senses your panic and, with his inhaler in the form teacher's desk, realises that he does not have effective help at hand. James has always felt embarrassed by his asthma, and so doesn't tell you what the problem is. James becomes increasingly anxious, which further exacerbates his asthma and so his breathing becomes even harder. Unsure of what to do, and not realising that James is having an asthma attack, you take him into the sick bay, lie him down, tuck him up with a thick blanket, and see how he gets on for a while.

Wrong!

When you are having an asthma attack you do not want to lie down. You want to expand your chest as much as possible. This is made easier by bracing the muscles in your rib cage, for which you need to be sitting up. Also, the blankets make it worse. Even the gentlest pressure on the chest feels massive, and makes it even more difficult to breathe.

James eventually tells you that he is asthmatic, and that he occasionally uses a blue inhaler. Another child is sent to collect James' inhaler from the other side of the school. By now James' distress and discomfort, coupled with lack of appropriate medication, will have worsened his attack so much that he will probably need to go to hospital.

Had the teacher been asthma-aware, he would have realised from the outset that James was having an asthma attack, and would have kept him calm by confidently taking charge of the situation. Just this action alone could have alleviated the attack. The teacher would then have taken James indoors, away from the cold air, sat him down quietly in a warm room, loosened the clothing around his chest and given him two or three puffs of his reliever medication. James would probably have made a full recovery within a few minutes. Better still, if James had had his inhaler in his pocket, he could have had a pre-exercise dose of reliever medication. The asthma attack would probably not have happened, and he could have participated fully in the game of football.

It is very likely that children will have asthma attacks at

school. After all, a school day is rife with many asthma triggers: exercise, stress, sudden temperature changes, grass pollen, tree pollen, fungi spores, animal fur, food allergies and, of course, coughs and colds.

Teachers must be informed about asthma. Asthma will be less of a burden to them if they are confident that they know how to deal with this potentially dangerous disease.

Creating A Favourable School Environment

In a favourable environment, nearly all asthma sufferers will be able to join in all normal school activities. To create such an environment, you need to increase asthma awareness in the school, advise teachers on how to recognise and deal with asthma, reduce asthma triggers in the school, and have a written School Asthma Protocol giving specific instructions on how to deal with asthma.

RAISING ASTHMA AWARENESS AT SCHOOL

Many asthmatics are embarrassed about their condition. They therefore hide their symptoms, and are reluctant to use their inhalers when they need to. This can lead to attacks occurring because the child does not inform someone that he is having difficulty breathing. Not using a reliever inhaler at the outset of an asthma attack can lead to a bad asthma attack.

Other children may regard asthma sufferers as being abnormal or different in some way, and therefore tease or bully them. This will make the asthma sufferer feel isolated, and thus more embarrassed and stigmatised by his condition. General awareness of asthma amongst parents, children and staff can go a long way towards overcoming these problems.

There are many methods of increasing asthma awareness. For instance, the children could do some fund-raising for an asthma charity, perhaps by doing a sponsored swim. If the asthmatic children in the school also participated in this, they could demonstrate that they do lead normal lives. This would be a good opportunity to put up display boards explaining the facts about asthma, and how the school aims to create a favourable environment for asthma sufferers.

Another idea is to invite the school doctor or local asthma nurse to give a talk to parents, staff and pupils. It would be very useful if one or two parents with asthma could talk about, and share their experiences.

The children might also enjoy doing a cross-curricular project on air, including asthma along with pollution, smells, germination, balloons, and so on. In this way asthma can be firmly positioned as part of life and, as such, not perceived as a stigma.

RECOGNISING ASTHMA

Children with undiagnosed asthma, or under-treated asthma, may have little more than a recurrent cough which may be more noticeable in the morning, or after exposure to an asthma trigger such as cold air or pollen. The child's sleep may be interrupted by asthma symptoms, so he may be tired and lacklustre the following day. Often, the only symptom a young child will complain of is a tightness in the chest.

An undiagnosed asthma sufferer, or an under-treated asthma sufferer, can lose up to 40 days schooling a year.

Physical education (PE) teachers are particularly well-placed to recognise a child with asthma. The asthmatic child may come up with various excuses to avoid PE lessons, or he may even absent himself from school on the day he has PE. Teachers should look out for a pattern in the absenteeism. During PE, he may be struggling to keep up with the other children, or may even be wheezing.

If you are teaching a child who has suspected asthma, or who is struggling with known asthma, discuss your concerns with the child's parents so that he can be assessed by his doctor.

SCREENING PUPILS FOR ASTHMA

The purpose of screening a school for asthma is to identify undiagnosed asthmatics, and to monitor the control of known asthmatics. The peak flows of all the children are noted before exercise. The children are then exercised vigorously for 6 minutes, and their peak flows recorded between 5 and 10 minutes after exercise. A drop of 15 per cent in the peak flow readings after exercise indicates a strong possibility of the child having asthma, or the child's asthma being poorly controlled. The child will then need to be assessed by his GP. Another way of screening for asthma is by using questionnaires which enquire after asthma symptoms such as coughing, wheezing and shortness of breath.

Screening schools for asthma using an exercise test is still experimental. If you are interested in screening your school for asthma, you must have the support of an asthma-aware and research-orientated doctor.

DEALING WITH AN ACUTE ATTACK

It is very important to recognise the early signs of an acute asthma attack so that appropriate steps can be promptly taken:

- The asthma sufferer often becomes quiet and withdrawn, struggling in the fight for breath.

- He will usually be wheezing (making a sound like a squeaky bagpipe) when he breathes out.

- He may sit with his hands pressed onto his knees, bracing the muscles in his upper body to assist his breathing.

- He may show recession (the indrawing of flesh above the sternum and between the ribs). This can be mimicked by placing a hand over your nose and mouth and trying to breathe in.

A *very dangerous situation* has developed when there is so little air going in and out of the lungs that:

- **The asthma sufferer cannot say more than one or two words.**

- **The wheeze disappears and the asthma sufferer becomes quiet. People often mistake this for the asthma sufferer improving; in fact he has become a lot worse.**

- **The recession becomes even more marked as the asthma sufferer desperately tries to suck air into his lungs.**

- **Ultimately the asthma sufferer starts to turn blue. This happens when insufficient oxygen reaches the tissues.**

If you are responsible for a child and have *any* suspicion that an acute asthma attack is developing, take prompt decisive action. This will be easier if your school has a written School Asthma Protocol. There is a suggested protocol on p. 160 that you can adapt for the specific needs of your own school. If you have a School Asthma Protocol, make sure you are familiar with it.

It must be stressed that there are around 2,000 asthma deaths in Britain each year, and a number of asthma sufferers die in the first hour of the attack. If you are responsible for a child who is experiencing an asthma attack, it is comforting to know that a few puffs of reliever could stop the attack there and then. The longer the attack goes on, the more difficult it becomes to treat.

Once you have recognised that the child is having an asthma attack, what should you do?

Firstly, allow the child to be involved. If he is a diagnosed asthmatic, it is his condition and he is used to it. If appropriate, use a peak flow meter.

Give the child a dose of his reliever. If the response is good and the wheezing subsides, you need take no further action, although it is essential to watch the child for any signs of wheeziness later on. **If a child does not have his own reliever handy he can use that of another child.** This conflicts with the usual advice given about not sharing medication. However, requiring reliever inhalers is one of the few times when it is quite acceptable and safe to use someone else's medicine.

If the child is having difficulty using his inhaler because his breathing is restricted, use a spacer device (see p. 47). This is far easier for him to use because there is no need for him to take a deep breath in. A spacer should always be kept readily available in a place specified in the School Asthma Protocol.

If only partial relief is obtained using the reliever inhaler, repeated dosages should be given until relief is obtained, or until medical assistance has arrived. If necessary, in an emergency situation, a whole canister of reliever medication can be used in this way. Effective treatment of asthma symptoms in schools has no hidden dangers, except that children who are using reliever inhalers can sometimes become twitchy and hyperactive after taking their medication. This state only lasts for a short while, and causes no lasting harm.

If the child is not getting quick and complete relief from his asthma symptoms after using a reliever inhaler, or if the symptoms return within four hours, then professional medical help is necessary. The urgency will of course depend on the child's condition, but, if in any doubt, seek urgent help from your school doctor, call an ambulance or take the child to your local casualty department. The course of action to be followed should be in your School Asthma Protocol.

REDUCING ASTHMA TRIGGERS AT SCHOOL

A number of simple measures can be adopted that will help all asthmatics, but will not unduly restrict children without asthma.

For example, many children are allergic to animals, and this may mean that rabbits, hamsters and mice cannot be kept in classrooms. Obviously, this should be handled very tactfully. The last thing an asthmatic child wants is to be branded as the killjoy who got rid of the much-loved pet. Alternatives can be found, such as keeping animals in an allocated 'pets corner' away from the classroom.

Teachers also need to watch the environmental conditions. The first few lungfuls of bitingly cold air that an asthmatic child takes in as she runs smartly from the warm changing room on to the playing field can trigger a serious attack. Similarly, trees and grass throw out millions of grains of pollen and tiny fungal spores into the air. They are suspended in the warm air that blows in and out of the classroom window, constantly threatening to trigger a primed airway. So be aware of the unseen dangers in the air, and encourage the asthma sufferer to use her reliever inhaler as soon as she experiences any asthma symptoms.

There are also man-made triggers in the air which are potentially harmful. Of these, traffic emissions and cigarette smoke are particularly potent, and should be avoided wherever possible.

Children who are old enough to handle their own medication should have their inhalers on them at all times. For small children, inhalers and spacers should always be readily available. It is crucial for children to be able to treat asthma symptoms immediately, and prevent their asthma from deteriorating.

Writing A School Asthma Protocol

It is important to have a protocol written down and generally available to teachers, parents and pupils, in order to ensure good asthma management in school. You may find that you need to adapt the following sample protocol in the light of circumstances specific to your school, or when there are new developments in asthma management.

General Principles

At *The Asthma Aware School*, we aim to consider fully the needs of asthmatic children. We will achieve this aim by ensuring our teaching staff are well informed about asthma. They will be able to recognise undiagnosed or inadequately treated asthmatics, and will be able to recognise and deal with an emergency situation.

Our pupils will also be asthma-aware in order to de-stigmatise the disease, encourage compliance with asthma treatment, and therefore enable the pupil to reach his full potential. We aim to promote individual responsibility for asthma self-management as early as possible.

Main Points

- The teaching staff receive regular training in the recognition and management of asthma, and other medical conditions relevant to the school environment.

- A record is kept of all known asthmatics, and their medication. It is updated each term.

- At an appropriate age, pupils are made aware of asthma, and other chronic illnesses, as a part of their general education and in order to destigmatise these diseases.

- Pupils carry their own inhalers as soon as they are able to assume this responsibility. For the younger pupils, their inhalers will be available wherever and whenever they are required.

- Spare reliever medication, spacer devices (the means for delivering this medication in an acute situation), and peak flow meters are located at convenient sites in the school.

- In acute asthma, reliever medication will be given to a child at the teacher's discretion. If necessary, repeated dosages will be given. Previously undiagnosed asthmatics will be managed in the same fashion. The school doctor will be informed immediately, and his advice on further management will be followed. If the doctor is not available, an ambulance will be called. The child's parents will also be informed immediately.

- If a child appears to be requiring reliever medication more than usual, the parent will be informed. The parent will also be informed if the child's asthma appears to be inadequately controlled.

- Pupils will be encouraged to have reliever medication available while playing sport. Spare reliever medication and a spacer device will always be at hand.

- It is the parents' responsibility to ensure that their child brings reliever medication on day-time school trips. For trips lasting more than a day, parents must ensure that their child also brings preventative medication.

- For young pupils who require preventative medication during the day, the form teacher will supervise administration, providing the parents give written instructions, and the pupil's medication is suitably labelled.

A School For Asthmatics

Pilgrims School, set at the top of cliffs overlooking the south coast of England, is for those very rare children whose asthma is difficult to control despite using maximum medication. For these children, their asthma (or eczema) is so bad it is literally ruining their lives. They will have missed weeks or months of schooling, and some may have spent up to half their lives in hospital. They may have emotional or behavioural problems because of their illness.

In order to be admitted to Pilgrims School a child must have a *Statement of Special Needs* from their local education authority. This is the body that will also be responsible for paying their fees. Since the school's fees are far higher than those at any other boarding school, the authorities are often reluctant to commit to sending a child there. Consequently, although the school can accommodate 56 children, there are usually a number of places unfilled. The very unwell asthmatic children who join Pilgrims School are in a sense the lucky ones, for soon after joining they all become very much better.

The school takes simple, commonsense measures for improving the environment for an asthmatic, and turns them into a disciplined science. There are no carpets; dust is sought out and zealously removed. In order to kill off house dust mites, all bedding, clothes and towels are boil-washed frequently. All chemicals used in cleaning materials have to be vetted. There are strict guidelines on diet, with each child having his or her own list of 'forbidden fruits'.

Despite the strict rules governing its environment, Pilgrims School is a happy place where children who have never felt able to join in sports go swimming daily, play football, go canoeing and join in all the normal activities they should have been able to join in when they lived at home.

Enabling the children to live a normal life involves a dedicated medical team providing 24-hour assistance. Each morning and evening every child visits Matron, who oversees the taking of medication. The doctor visits three times a week, there is an annual examination by the paediatrician, and as soon as any child shows signs of having problems with their asthma they are taken to the medical wing to be looked after. Recovery tends to be swift: the child is motivated to recover so as to be able to resume his or her activities.

This approach works. It is now several years since any child from Pilgrims has had to be admitted to hospital.

The environment is controlled, all the latest equipment is available, and because their asthma is correctly treated the children tend not to get ill while they are at school. The school also helps pupils to manage their asthma when they are at home.

One of the first tasks for the school doctor is to release new pupils from what is known as the asthma trap. This happens when a child has been prescribed asthma drug after asthma drug by their doctor, or hospital, or both.

Each time a new prescription was issued scant concern was paid to the number of drugs the child was already taking, what good they were doing, and how all those drugs might interact.

The school doctor usually cuts the drug intake of new pupils quite severely, paring away the unnecessary medications. Those that remain must be taken strictly according to instructions.

Pilgrims School has an impressive success rate, with many of its pupils gaining A levels and going on to further education. But its real success can be measured not in its exam results but in the fact that it enables pupils to lead ordinary lives. When you are a child who has been in and out of hospital and school, and who arrives with a supply of 12 or more different prescribed asthma medications, being 'ordinary' is very important.

13

ASTHMA AND POLLUTION

Our bodies are superbly adapted to live in the mantle of air that surrounds our planet. We need a continuous supply of oxygen (O_2), which is extracted from the air by our lungs, and exchanged for carbon dioxide (CO_2). Plants, trees and algae absorb CO_2 and, using power from the rays of the sun, return oxygen back to the air.

What Causes Air Pollution?

Too often, we take this great natural system, which has taken millions of years to evolve, and is still evolving, very much for granted. We are only too willing to use air as a waste disposal unit for power station emissions and car exhaust. Because we are unable to see most of the pollutants we put into the air, we are generally complacent about air quality. Yet surely it is just as socially unacceptable to litter the air as it is to litter the streets? One of the main reasons for not leaving litter in our streets is that it encourages the spread of disease. Yet we now know that litter in the air (pollution) causes illness and death just as surely as any epidemic. Historians will look back in horror at the 'Great 100 Year Pollution Epidemic'.

INDUSTRIAL AIR POLLUTION

Man's ability to generate major air pollution began with the Industrial Revolution. Coal kept the wheels of industry turning. When coal burns it produces two main pollutants: sulphur dioxide (SO_2) and particulates. When SO_2 is inhaled, it combines with moisture on the surface of the airways, forming sulphuric acid (H_2SO_4). Experiments have shown that exposing asthmatics to increasing concentrations of SO_2 causes a corresponding increase in asthma symptoms. H_2SO_4 forming inside the airways is clearly highly irritating to the airways, and in primed airways can trigger an asthma attack.

Particulates are very fine particles formed primarily of organic material. Particulates of less than 10 microns in diameter are particularly dangerous, as they can go right into the lungs. SO_2 combines with moisture on the surface of particulates, forming H_2SO_4, which is then carried deep into the lungs. Together, SO_2 and particulates produce a greater effect than they would acting separately.

ACID RAIN

Acid rain is formed by SO_2 and oxides of nitrogen (NO_x) combining with moisture in the air to form H_2SO_4 and nitric acid (HNO_3). These acids devastate the trees and plants that play a vital role in maintaining the oxygen in the air we breathe. Up to 60 per cent of trees in industrial areas are damaged by acid rain.

It is the combination of particulates and SO_2 that produces the acrid 'pea soup' smogs that have hung over the industrial areas of the world for the past 100 years. The London smog of 1952 caused 4,000 deaths in one month, mainly from 'chest problems'. This led to the Clean Air Act of 1956. Only smokeless fuels could be burnt in urban areas, and there was a high chimney policy in order to disperse the pollutants more effectively into the air.

MOTOR VEHICLE POLLUTION

Since the London smog, the pattern of pollution has changed. There has been a steady decline in pollution from burning coal in power stations and heavy industry. But this has been counterbalanced by the huge increase in the numbers of vehicles on the road, and in the pollution they produce. Along with this increase in motor vehicle pollution, there has been a dramatic increase in asthma.

> In Southern Ontario, Canada, the reasons people were admitted into 79 hospitals were recorded. Information was also collected from nearby pollution sampling stations. The reasons for hospital admission and the pollution data were then analysed. Statistically significant associations were found for hospital admission and SO_2 and ozone (O_3) levels.

The main pollutants produced by petrol vehicles are oxides of nitrogen (NO_x) and SO_2. Diesel vehicles, which until recently were thought of as being reasonably 'clean', produce particulates that are now known to be important pollutants. NO_x, like SO_2, combines with moisture on the surface of the airways to produce nitric acid (HNO_3). This is highly irritating to the airways, and experiments have clearly shown that NO_x can produce asthma symptoms in known asthmatics. NO_x also appears to inhibit the defences of the airways, making viral infections more likely. As we have already seen, the rhinovirus is the most common trigger for asthma; it appears to act together with NO_x, their combined effect being greater than each would have separately.

IN-CAR POLLUTION

Experiments in the USA and Europe have shown that in-car pollution can be tenfold higher than the pollution level outside a car. This is because exhaust fumes are drawn into the car through the air intake vents but do not escape so readily, particularly if the windows are closed.

PHOTOCHEMICAL SMOG

NO_x interacts with particulates and sunlight to form another highly reactive chemical compound called ozone (O_3). High up in our atmosphere, ozone protects us from the harmful ultraviolet rays in sunlight. But at ground level, ozone is a highly reactive compound which is a potent irritant to the airways. This *photochemical pollution* requires sunlight to provide the necessary energy for the chemical pollutants to interact to form ozone. This leads to the familiar photochemical haze that can frequently be seen on a warm summer's day.

Photochemical smog is likely to form in places with still air, bright sunlight, and a high concentration of motor vehicles. Los Angeles is the world's blackspot for this type of smog. The Los Angeles basin is formed by hills on three sides, and the sea on the fourth, trapping the air and producing low wind speeds. There is a very high density of motor vehicles, and a warm sunny climate.

In Britain, photochemical smog forms when there is an anticyclone (high pressure system), characterised by warm sunny weather above the country, accompanied by a temperature inversion (a layer of cold air at ground level, with warm air above). This prevents the pollutants being dispersed by convection (normally ground-level, warm air rises), effectively trapping pollutants at ground level. Britain's worst episode of photochemical smog occurred in 1976, when visibility at Heathrow Airport was reduced to just 2 kilometres.

Would Reducing Air Pollution Really Help?

Air pollutants clearly act as trigger factors for asthma. The ongoing debate centres around whether or not air pollution can act as an initiator of asthma. This would be difficult to demonstrate scientifically, as it would be almost impossible to protect people entirely from other potential initiators such as different pollens or house dust mites.

However, we *do* know that pollutants are potent triggers of asthma, and that most triggers can also act as initiators. Furthermore, since it is generally agreed that the massive rise in asthma mirrors the increase in pollution due to road vehicle emissions, it is highly likely that these pollutants act as initiators, as well as triggers, for asthma.

Air pollution is particularly likely to initiate asthma in children because:

- NO_x inhibits the defence mechanisms of the airways, making children more susceptible to viral infections, such as the very common rhinovirus.

- A three-year-old child breathes in twice as much air per unit of body weight as an adult.

- Children spend a lot of time running around outdoors and therefore inhale large quantities of polluted air.

What Can We Do About Pollution?

AS INDIVIDUALS

In Britain, the Air Quality Bulletins relate to the levels of NO_x, SO_2 and O_3 in the air. The air quality is divided into four bands: very good, good, poor and very poor. This information is included in most weather reports on television, radio, in newspapers and also on CEEFAX. Each country has its equivalent.

When the air quality is in the poor and very poor bands it is advisable for asthma sufferers to increase their preventative medication until the air quality improves. This applies particularly to asthma sufferers who know that poor air quality triggers their asthma. The air quality for an area may be reported as being good, but there can be isolated pockets of poor quality air. If you can, you need to both see and smell the quality of the air. If there are high levels of O_3 and particulates there will be a haze. If you can smell car exhausts then there will be high levels of NO_x.

When the air quality is very poor, unless your asthma is quite brittle and you are particularly sensitive to pollution, it is generally unnecessary to seal yourself in your house or office by closing all the windows and doors. However, it is best to avoid exerting yourself, for instance by jogging, so as not to inhale large amounts of polluted air.

As A Community

As a community, we need to reduce pollution as much and as quickly as we can. Ultimately, we must aim to be as close to a non-polluting society as possible. With determination, we could go a long way towards achieving the following goals over the next 20 years:

- **To have catalytic converters on all cars:** Catalytic converters reduce polluting emissions by 90 per cent but they increase fuel consumption by 3–9 per cent and are not effective for journeys under 5 miles. That represents two-thirds of all car journeys. Overall, they are beneficial, but the best conversion would be to non-polluting cars.

  Where there are significant risks of damage to the environment, the government will be prepared to take precautionary action . . . even where scientific knowledge is not conclusive.
  'This common inheritance', Department of the
  Environment White Paper, 1992

- **To produce motor vehicles that cause minimal pollution:** The internal combustion engine can be modified to run as a minimal polluter by using natural gas as the source of fuel. The only waste products are water and CO_2. There are already about 1 million natural gas vehicles worldwide.

Another way of making an internal combustion engine effectively a minimal polluter has recently been developed. The car radiator is coated with a special precious metal coating. During the journey the coating is heated by the radiator. As air passes over this coating, NO_x and O_3 react together, eliminating both pollutants. Using this system, the car can actually eliminate more NO_x than it produces.

Electric cars are in an advanced stage of development. Used in busy urban areas, electric cars remove pollution from populated areas. However, the electricity has to be produced in a power station. If this is an old inefficient coal fired station, overall electrically powered cars could add to pollution.

The first electric bus service in the world has gone into operation in Luxemburg. The buses have special quick-charge batteries that can be boosted to 40 per cent capacity in only 12 minutes. This means the buses can be operated almost continuously during the day, stopping only briefly at special fast-charge facilities in the city.

- **To change the way we travel, placing more emphasis on public transport, walking, cycling and park-and-ride schemes:** Attracting more people on to public transport would require considerable investment and would need the political will to do so, as well as substantial government subsidies.

- **To make fossil fuel power stations as 'clean' as possible:** Fossil fuel burning power stations can already be made considerably cleaner by installing desulphurisation equipment which removes the harmful SO_2 emissions. Every power station should be fitted with this equipment.

- **To develop and invest in alternative sources of non-polluting power:** These are schemes that produce power from sources such as the wind, hydroelectricity and from the waves. These can, however, have a major detrimental impact on the environment. Hydroelectric schemes often involve building huge dams that have wide ranging environmental implications. Wind farms need unsightly wind turbines placed over a large area. Removing power from the waves may cause considerable damage to coastal life that needs the constant movement of water to provide O_2 and nutrients.

- **To invest heavily in the development of fusion power stations:** At present, nuclear power stations produce power by splitting the atom. This produces hazardous nuclear waste. Fusion power stations produce power by pushing atoms together, and would not produce any radioactive waste, nor any other pollutants. It is possible that fusion power will be available by the early part of the next century. This, together with electrically powered cars, would vastly reduce the level of air pollution.

The fact that it will be difficult to get hard information on the long-term effects of air pollution on health should not be used to delay action on trying to reduce current levels of pollution.
Chair, Department of Heath Advisory Group, 1992

14

HAYFEVER, ECZEMA AND ALLERGIES

The Atopic Tendency

Allergens are common trigger factors for asthma. The most common asthma-triggering allergen is the faeces of the house dust mite. Some asthma sufferers are allergic to particular pollens and only experience asthma at certain times of the year. If asthma is triggered by an allergen as opposed to an irritant, the asthma sufferer is said to have an atopic tendency.

This means that the person is genetically predisposed to suffer with allergic problems generally. The two conditions that are most closely associated with asthma in this context are eczema and hayfever. In families that have an atopic tendency, different family members may have eczema, hayfever or asthma. Some unlucky people suffer from all three conditions at the same time.

What Do Hayfever, Eczema And Asthma Have In Common?

Hayfever, eczema and asthma share many features. For example, they may all be triggered by both allergens and irritants (hayfever-like symptoms triggered by an irritant are called rhinitis). Once triggered, the response is inappropriate inflammation, the effects of which depend on the site of inflammation.

Eczema is an inflammation in the skin, so there is redness, swelling and cracking of the skin. Hayfever is an inflammation in the lining of the nose and surface layer of the eyes (conjunctivae), so there is redness and swelling of the lining of the nose and the conjunctivae. Asthma is an inflammation in the lining of the airways, so there is redness and swelling in the airways, causing them to become narrowed.

The treatment for all three conditions is in many respects also similar, aiming to control the underlying inflammation. For mild eczema, simple moisturising creams and bath oils may be sufficient. If the eczema is more severe, a short period of a steroid cream, such as hydrocortisone, may be necessary. These must always be used under a doctor's supervision as long-term use of steroid creams can cause thinning of the skin, particularly on the face. For hayfever, antihistamine tablets may be sufficient. If not, the anti-inflammatory medicine Opticrom (cromoglycate) can be

---

HISTAMINE AND ANTI-HISTAMINES

Chemicals called inflammatory mediators accumulate at the site of inflammation, and help to increase the inflammation. Histamine is one of these inflammatory mediators. Anti-histamines block the actions of histamine, and are effective in controlling hayfever.

Although histamine is an inflammatory mediator in asthma, anti-histamines are unfortunately not an effective treatment for asthma.

---

delivered as eye or nose drops, or there are steroid sprays for the nose.

Other Allergies

People with an atopic tendency are also more likely to suffer from other allergies, such as contact allergies to particular metals in jewellery (nickel is a common allergen), causing inflammation in the skin. Just about every substance has caused an allergic reaction in someone at some time. Common culprits are detergents, scented soaps and make-up.

LIFE-THREATENING ALLERGIC REACTIONS

Severe life-threatening allergic reactions are known as ana-phylactic reactions. People with an atopic tendency are pre-disposed to develop anaphylactic reactions. These reactions occur without warning, and can be provoked by a factor that has never previously caused a problem for that person. Common allergens which cause anaphylactic reactions are wasp stings and peanuts. In the UK about five people a year die from wasp stings.

In an anaphylactic reaction, inflammation can occur gen-erally throughout the body, often first becoming apparent with a swollen tongue and weals on the skin. However, the main danger comes from swelling inflammation in the air-ways which is like a very severe asthma attack. Death is usu-ally due to a respiratory arrest (insufficient oxygen getting through to the blood).

The treatment for anaphylaxis is injected adrenaline. This acts to open up the airways, in the same way as adrenaline-like reliever medication is used in asthma. It is important that an anaphylactic reaction is treated promptly, and often with repeated doses of adrenaline.

If a person has previously had an anaphylactic reaction to an allergen to which they could easily be exposed again, for example a wasp sting, they should discuss with their doctor whether they need to carry adrenaline.

GLOSSARY

ACUTE
Sudden and very serious. An acute asthma attack is dangerous and can be life-threatening.

ADD-ON MEDICATIONS
In asthma these medications are used *in addition to* reliever and preventer medications.

ADRENALINE
A hormone produced by the body in response to stress. In asthma it has the effect of relaxing the muscles surrounding the airways.

ALLERGEN
In asthma, an allergen is a substance in our environment which the body mistakenly believes to be harmful. When the body encounters an allergen it responds with an inappropriate inflammatory response.

ALLOPATHIC TREATMENT
Another name for conventional medical treatment, which is based on the principal of treating disease with opposition.

ALVEOLI
Air-filled sacs at the end of the bronchioles.

ANAPHYLAXIS
Severe, life-threatening allergic reactions.

ASTHMA MANAGEMENT PLAN
A system for managing asthma which is drawn up by the asthma sufferer in partnership with a doctor or asthma nurse. The plan will help you monitor your asthma and adjust your medication to meet changing demands. It also includes simple measures you can take to reduce your exposure to triggers, and a plan of action if you require emergency medical assistance. It is important that your Asthma Management Plan is tailored to meet your own needs.

ATOPIC TENDENCY
If a person's body contains genes which predispose them to develop allergies, they are said to have an atopic tendency.

BEHAVIOURAL THERAPY
In asthma, behavioural therapy is used to assist the asthmatic in coping with the situations that cause asthma-triggered panic attacks. It involves teaching techniques

for dealing with the feared situation, and should only be undertaken under the guidance of a professional therapist.

BRITTLE ASTHMA
A very unpredictable and severe form of asthma.

BRONCHI
The two main branches of the trachea.

BRONCHIOLES
Small sub-divisions of the bronchial tubes.

BRONCHITIS
A chronic infection of the medium-sized airways, often leading to breathing difficulties.

CHROMOSOME
Formed by long chains of genes and other genetic material. Every cell in the body has 46 chromosomes, apart from sperm and eggs which have half of this number.

COGNITIVE THERAPY
A psychological treatment which can help asthma sufferers who are having episodes of panic caused by the stress and fear of having asthma.

COMPLIANCE
Understanding why you need your medication, and taking it regularly as prescribed.

CORTICOSTEROID
Medications containing anti-inflammatory agents called steroids. In asthma they are used as a preventative medication.

COUNSELLING
In asthma, counselling may help a depressed asthmatic to resolve the problems that are causing his depression.

CROUP
Croup is a condition caused by a viral infection of the large upper airways. It produces a harsh sound during inhalation, and a barking cough.

CYANOSIS
A feature that occurs when there is too little oxygen in the blood. In cyanosis the lips and tongue turn grey or blue.

DANDER
Dead flakes of animal skin.

DENIAL
A pattern of behaviour in which people refuse to admit the reality or existence of something. Some asthmatics deny that they are ill, and refuse to take their medication because this would mean admitting that they were ill.

DEPRESSION
A depressed mood is characterised by extreme gloom, feelings of inadequacy and inability to concentrate. Depression is a known asthma trigger, and asthma is thought to increase existing depression.

DRY POWDER INHALER (DPI)
A type of inhaler used to deliver asthma medication. The medication is released in the form of a dry powder.

GLOSSARY

ECZEMA
Inflammation of the skin, causing redness, swelling and cracking. Like asthma, eczema can be triggered by allergens or irritants.

EMPHYSEMA
The alveolar region of the lung is damaged, forming dilated sacs that become chronically infected. This results in a cough and shortness of breath.

EXCLUSION DIET
A method of investigating whether certain foods are asthma triggers. Under an exclusion diet, most foods, except for a few basics, are eliminated and then re-introduced to the diet under controlled conditions. The exclusion diet is explained fully on page 68.

FAMILY THERAPY
A way of helping a family to deal with their interactive problems, such as communication, or over-protectiveness. Family therapy can help the family to manage an individual's asthma, and to cope with the effects of that asthma.

FOOD ADDITIVES
Substances used to preserve or enhance food. Food additives can exacerbate asthma in a small number of asthmatics. In Europe these additives must be listed on food packaging.

GENE
The basic unit of heredity. Genes determine your physical characteristics. It is the combination of your genes and your interaction with the environment which determines whether you will develop asthma, and how severe it will be.

GENERIC
The generic name is the name given to the basic chemical compound of a medication.

HAYFEVER
An inflammation in the lining of the nose and surface layer of the eyes.

HYPERVENTILATION
The condition in which a person *overbreathes* (breathes deeper and faster than usual), often as a result of a panic attack.

INITIATOR
The factor that starts up the underlying inflammation in the airways of an asthmatic.

IRRITANT
A substance in our environment which can harm our body. When our body encounters an irritant it defends itself with an appropriate inflammatory response.

LUMEN
The hollow part of the airways.

METERED DOSE INHALER (MDI)
A type of inhaler, and the most commonly used delivery system for asthma medication. An MDI is a metal canister encased in a plastic shell. The medication is released in the form of an aerosol spray.

NEBULISER
A system for delivering asthma medication via a face mask. It is particularly useful for children. The mask is placed over the face, and attached to the nebuliser which generates a fine mist containing the asthma medication. The asthmatic inhales the medication via normal breathing.

OCCUPATIONAL ASTHMA
Asthma which is initiated and/or triggered by factors in the workplace.

PANIC ATTACK
An episode of acute anxiety in which the heart beats rapidly and sweating occurs. It is usually accompanied by hyperventilation.

PANIC DISORDER
A condition that features recurrent, brief panic attacks.

PEAK FLOW METER
A device for measuring the speed at which air comes out of the lungs. It is used for self-monitoring of asthma.

PREVENTATIVE MEDICATION
The mainstay of good asthma management. Preventative medication uses inhaled corticosteroids to control the underlying inflammation in the lungs, and so lessen the likelihood of an asthma attack. The containers for inhaled preventative medicine are always coloured either light brown, dark brown, maroon or orange.

PRIMED
In asthma, constant low-grade inflammation in the airways makes the lining of the airways unstable or *primed*, and hyper-reactive to particularly hostile factors called triggers.

PSYCHOLOGY
The study of human and animal behaviour. Psychological factors such as depression, panic and excessive emotion have an effect on asthma.

RECESSION
Drawing in of the flesh between the ribs and above the sternum (breastbone). Recession occurs in someone who is experiencing severe breathing difficulties.

RELIEVER MEDICATION
Relievers are inhaled from blue containers, and are used to treat asthma symptoms such as wheezing, coughing and shortness of breath. Also called bronchodilators, relievers contain an adrenaline-like medication which relaxes the muscles surrounding the airways. Relievers are not anti-inflammatory. Sometimes they are prescribed orally in tablet or syrup form.

RHINITIS
Hayfever-like symptoms triggered by an irritant.

SCREENING
A way of identifying undiagnosed asthmatics. Screening in schools is described on page 156.

TRACHEA
The tube which takes air from the larynx to the bronchi. Its non-technical name is windpipe.

TRIGGER
There are numerous factors which provoke asthma attacks in people with established asthma. Any of these factors is called a trigger.

WHEEZING
An involuntary sound made by an asthmatic when breathing out. Wheezing can sound like a feeble bagpipe, or a multi-toned whistle.

USEFUL ADDRESSES

UK

British Lung Foundation
New Garden House
78 Hatton Garden
London EC1N 8JR

National Asthma Campaign
Providence House
Providence Place
London N1 0NT

**National Asthma Training
Centre**
Winton House
Church Street
Stratford-upon-Avon
Warwickshire CV37 6HB

The Sports Council
Doping Control Unit
Walkden House
3–10 Melton Street
London NW1 2EB

Pilgrims School
Firle Road
Seaford
East Sussex BN25 2HX

**Institute for
Complementary Medicine**
PO Box 194
London SE16 1QZ

**The British Acupuncture
Association**
34 Alderney Street
London SW1

**The Society of Teachers of
the Alexander Technique**
20 London House
266 Fulham Road
London SW10 9EL

**The London College of
Classical Homoeopathy**
Morley College
61 Westminster Bridge Road
London SE1 7HT

The Society of Homoeopaths
2 Artizan Road
Northampton NN1 4HU

**British Society of
Hypnotherapists**
37 Orbain Road
Fulham
London SW6 7JZ

The National Institute of Medical Herbalists
56 Longbrook Street
Exeter
Devon EX4 6AH

The Association of Reflexologists
27 Old Gloucester Street
London WC1N 3XX

AUSTRALIA

Asthma Australia
(Australian Association of Asthma Foundations)
PO Box 360
Woden A.C.T. 2606

National Asthma Campaign
615 St Kilda Road
Melbourne
Victoria 3004

NEW ZEALAND

Asthma Foundation of New Zealand
PO Box 96–025
Balmoral
Auckland 3

SOUTH AFRICA

Mrs P E Bird
508 Savoy Apartments
183 Berea Road
Durban 4001

USA

Allergy and Asthma Network
Mothers of Asthmatics, Inc.
3554 Chainbridge Road
Suite 200
Fairfax
Virginia 22030–2709

The Asthma and Allergy Foundation of America
1125 15th Street, NW #502
Washington DC 20005

The American Lung Association
1740 Broadway
New York 10019–4374

CANADA

Allergy Asthma Information Association
#10, 65 Tromley Drive
Etobicoke
Ontario
M9B 5Y7

Canadian Lung Association
75 Albert Street
Ottawa
Ontario

Asthma Society of Canada
130 Bridgeland Avenue
Suite 425
Toronto
Ontario

INDEX

185